What

Top-Performing

Healthcare

Organizations

Know

What
Top-Performing
Healthcare
Organizations
Know

7 Proven Steps for Accelerating and Achieving Change

Greg Butler and Chip Caldwell

ACHE Management Series

Your board, staff, or clients may also benefit from this book's insight. For more information on quantity discounts, contact the Health Administration Press Marketing Manager at (312) 424-9470.

14 13 12 11 10 09   5 4 3 2 1

Butler, Greg.
  What top-performing healthcare organizations know : 7 proven steps for accelerating and achieving change / Greg Butler and Chip Caldwell.
      p. ; cm.
  Includes bibliographical references and index.
  ISBN-13: 978-1-56793-302-4 (alk. paper)
  ISBN-10: 1-56793-302-5 (alk. paper)
  1. Health facilities—Administration. 2. Public health administration. 3. Organizational change. I. Caldwell, Chip. II. Title.
  [DNLM: 1. Health Facilities—organization & administration. 2. Efficiency, Organizational. 3. Organizational Innovation. 4. Quality Assurance, Health Care—methods. WX 27.1 B985w 2009]
  RA971.B897 2009
  362.1068—dc22

                                    2008022617

The paper used in this publication meets the minimum requirements of American National Standard for Information Sciences-Permanence of Paper for Printed Library Materials, ANSI Z39.48-1984. ∞ ™

Project manager: Jennifer Seibert; Acquisitions editor: Janet Davis; Book designer: Scott R. Miller; Printer: Data Reproductions

Health Administration Press
A division of the Foundation
  of the American College of
  Healthcare Executives
One North Franklin Street
Suite 1700
Chicago, IL 60606
(312) 424-2800

Contents

DATE DUE

Acknowledgments

WE WOULD LIKE to acknowledge the individuals and organizations who have contributed to the development of the ideas, concepts, methods, and case studies in this book. These individuals' commitment to improve healthcare delivery has inspired us and furthered our learning process.

We especially would like to thank Lynne Sisak, Mike Brown, John Grah, and Bruce Tilley of Chip Caldwell and Associates for their pioneering work in uncovering the critical ideas that evolved into the in-quality staffing concept. Their work resulted in the development of proven methods for transforming healthcare data into actionable information. Their collective experience in hospital operations created solutions for eliminating common constraints that negatively affect patient care and throughput in the U.S. healthcare system.

We also wish to acknowledge Sherry Bright, formerly of Chip Caldwell and Associates, for her innovative work in piloting and formalizing the 100-Day Quality Workout approach for change acceleration. In addition, contributions by Tom Day and his team at HMC in constructing the initial framework for the quantum improver analysis in 2004 brought insight and statistical evidence to our initial findings. Finally, we would like to acknowledge Nancy Poston, senior vice president, Erlanger Health System, for her content and editorial assistance.

Preface

IN HIS BEST-SELLING BOOK *Good to Great: Why Some Companies Make the Leap...and Others Don't*, Jim Collins (2001) examined 1,435 "good" companies and analyzed how and why 11 of those companies became "great," isolating attributes that contributed to success. From his research, Collins concluded that every organization could inspire its own "pocket of greatness." Although his book targeted business leaders, the concept of studying successful organizations and determining what makes them successful is intriguing when applied to healthcare organizations.

In 2003 and 2004, we at Caldwell and Associates, LLC, collaborated with other healthcare leaders to take an in-depth look at the healthcare industry in terms of the premise and design of Collins's work (Pieper 2004). Some of the questions posed by our study were the same as those proposed by Collins, and others were unique to healthcare. What separates hospitals that demonstrate consecutive years of performance improvement from hospitals that have failed to achieve lasting gains? How do great hospitals formulate strategies, use benchmarks, set goals, and achieve tangible results? Are these differentiators transferable from one healthcare organization to another? Can these differentiators be isolated and replicated? How do they relate to the use of advanced quality methods such as Lean and Six Sigma?

DESIGN OF GOOD-TO-BEST RESEARCH

To answer these critical questions, we partnered with HMC of Boston, a leading comparative data company, and studied 222 hospitals with capacities ranging from 15 to 854 beds. For each organization, we measured the percentage change in cost per case mix-adjusted discharge from 2001 to 2002. We named organizations that ranked in the 75th percentile or higher "quantum improvers" and designated those in the bottom quartile as "nonstarters" (Pieper 2004). The research team interviewed executives and decision support staff within these two groups. The team did not inform participants whether their hospitals were in the quantum improver group or in the nonstarter group.

In the five years since we started conducting our research, we have continued to examine healthcare organizations and their work. We are currently in the early stages of the next generation of research. We have taken the attributes identified in earlier research and developed an assessment tool that measures 57 variables related to an organization's structure, culture, and use of quality acceleration methods. Our belief is that these attributes and elements are predictive of an organization's ability to transform its work processes successfully.

From our research, we gleaned characteristics of quantum improvers that contribute significantly to their success. Likewise, we identified characteristics and behaviors of nonstarter organizations that contribute toward their lack of progress.

The theories and recommendations in this book are based on attributes identified by our research and tested across a broad spectrum of healthcare settings. The book's main premise proposes that an organization's success hinges on how transformational initiatives are organized for accountability and action. In other words, structure drives culture as much as culture drives structure. On the basis of this research and professional experience, we developed a model that healthcare organizations can use to organize transformation efforts. This book introduces that model and provides organizations with a step-by-step approach to implementing performance improvement projects.

CONTENT OF THE BOOK

In Chapter 1, we discuss why change is necessary in healthcare and why many organizations struggle with it. This chapter provides a foundation for our work and addresses the critical role the senior leader plays in achieving transformational change.

Chapter 2 outlines our research and describes the differences between quantum improver organizations and nonstarter organizations. We also present our model for improvement in this chapter, which provides the basis for the following four chapters. Each chapter discusses one of the four main components of the model:

• Organizing for accountability
• Linking strategy to quality
• Creating an environment for change
• Using advanced quality methods

The final chapter transforms our model into a seven-step process organizations can use to design and implement performance improvement initiatives.

This book is not a rehash of technical material on advanced quality methods contained in manuals that already exist in healthcare literature, nor is it a "how to" guide for quality professionals on advanced quality methods such as Lean methodology and Six Sigma. This book was written for senior leaders and performance improvement professionals who wish to master the art of managing change and innovation. It provides quality professionals, financial analysts, Six Sigma black belts, department managers, and physician leaders with a context and plan to synergize their roles with the strategic mind-set of senior leaders.

Over the last decade, little evidence exists that healthcare leaders have been able to corral the complexities of healthcare to drive change. Although well intentioned, many senior leaders have not been able to achieve and sustain performance improvement and operational success. The seven-step process presented in this book can help senior leaders drive change, realize improvement, and transform their organizations from good to great.

REFERENCES

Collins, J. 2001. *Good to Great: Why Some Companies Make the Leap...and Others Don't.* New York: Harper Collins Publishing.

Pieper, S. 2004. "'Good to Great' in Healthcare: How Some Organizations Are Elevating Their Performance." *Healthcare Executive* 19 (4): 20–26.

CHAPTER 1

The Need for Change and
Why It Isn't Happening

There is nothing permanent except change.

—Heraclitus (540–475 B.C.)

CHANGE IS ONE of the few constants in our existence, permeating every element of our daily experience. The world around us is changing at an ever-increasing pace. We live in "exponential times."

Contrast yesterday to a day in your life a decade ago. Yesterday, you began your day receiving news that streamed in real time across your personal digital assistant. You listened to your MP3 player while you made breakfast and placed a few phone calls from your car using your hands-free Bluetooth device. None of these technologies existed ten years ago. Your car contains more computational power and information technology than NASA's most advanced spacecraft of the 1970s, and the number of communications you will receive today probably will exceed all the communication you received in an entire week only a few years ago.

The information age has brought us unprecedented access to information and exponential growth in computing speed and data storage. Experts predict that each of these factors will continue to double every 18 months. Our ability to connect to the Internet is becoming ubiquitous, creating expectations that information should be instantly accessible from any point on Earth. The Internet is rapidly transforming the way people learn, interact, and conduct daily business, and undoubtedly it will continue to play an increasingly critical role in all aspects of our lives, including healthcare.

Change has affected the workforce as well. One out of four employees has been employed with his or her company for less than one year, and employment experts estimate that today's careerist will work for 10 to 14 employers in his or her lifetime. U.S. Secretary of Education Richard Riley stated in a recent speech "that the top 10 jobs of 2010 are jobs that didn't even exist in 2004" (Fisch and McLeod 2007). The implications of these facts are profound. Current students are preparing to work for companies that do not exist today, to use technologies that have yet to be created, and to solve issues we have not yet identified as problems.

WHY CHANGE IS NECESSARY IN HEALTHCARE

Healthcare is not immune to the current velocity of change and the mega-trends shaping our society. In addition, healthcare faces its own unique issues. Today's senior healthcare executives must contend with an endless parade of challenges that keep their organizations in a constant state of flux. The following issues are a few of the major forces affecting healthcare.

- *Mounting pressures to reduce healthcare spending.* Any set of statistics clearly shows that the growth trends in U.S. healthcare expenditures are not sustainable. Currently, the United States spends significantly more on healthcare in total dollars and as a percentage of the gross domestic product (GDP) than does any other industrialized nation (Anderson 2000). According to the Centers for Medicare & Medicaid Services (CMS), healthcare has become the largest segment of the U.S. economy, representing approximately $2.2 trillion dollars, or 16.5 percent of the GDP (Baker 2007). Estimates from CMS

(Baker 2007) and the World Health Organization (2000) project that U.S. national healthcare spending will reach 20 percent of the GDP by 2015 without significant changes to the healthcare system.

- *Evolving consumer attitudes and expectations.* A quick scan of any newspaper confirms that consumers' attitudes and views about healthcare are changing rapidly. Unfortunately, most opinion polls indicate that this change is not for the better. The public is fed a steady diet of negative stories reinforcing the notion that healthcare is, at best, bureaucratic, bloated, unsafe, and inefficient and, at worst, greedy, corrupt, and run for the sole benefit of providers and payers.

  At the same time, today's consumers have come to expect more from their healthcare. They are better informed and no longer rely on their physicians as their sole source of information. Extensive information on diseases and treatment options is instantly available over the Internet, and the web can quickly link people with similar health interests around the globe. For example, a patient in Idaho can complete an online assessment that a physician in Alabama will review for a prescription that will be shipped from Canada. Someone with a rare medical condition can instantly contact thousands of patients suffering the same affliction. In addition, an abundance of information on alternatives to traditional medicine is available, and information on new medical procedures and breakthroughs flows directly to healthcare consumers, unfiltered by traditional medical review.

- *Transparency of quality outcomes.* Recent advances in Internet-based communications, new public accountability agencies, and current political agendas have raised the bar on availability of consumer-based healthcare quality indicators. Many organizations, such as Erlanger Health System in Chattanooga, Tennessee, have begun posting quality indicators on their websites for public review, allowing patients to compare and contrast the quality of different healthcare organizations. This transparency of quality outcomes may be problematic for academic medical centers that traditionally have based their reputations for quality on the "teaching" halo. Although important, teaching status may affect quality indicators negatively because some staff members are still learning how to provide effective healthcare. Unfortunately, consumer-accepted quality metrics will dwarf the benefits of a teaching hospital before the end of this decade.

- *Changing demographics and an aging population.* The world's population is growing at an unprecedented rate. Although the planet's population did not reach 1 billion until the 1850s, the U.S. Census Bureau (2000) is projecting the worldwide population to exceed 10 billion by 2040. The population of the United States alone has increased threefold between 1900 and 2000.

  The droves of baby boomer retirees headed for Medicare are just beginning. By 2020, the number of seniors in the United States is expected to exceed 55 million. It will reach 80 million by 2040. In contrast, birthrates in Western industrialized countries, including the United States, continue to fall, whereas birthrates in other parts of the world continue to grow.

  These demographic shifts will have a profound effect on healthcare. They will alter the clinical case mix of every hospital and the available talent pool from which healthcare providers recruit staff. Seismic shifts in immigration and ethnic backgrounds will alter the mix of services required by the communities that healthcare organizations serve and will result in significant changes ranging from the type of facilities built to the methods of delivering care.

- *Expanding treatment options.* Hospitals are not the sole providers of healthcare anymore. In recent years, technology growth and consumer demand have spawned a host of stand-alone surgical centers, specialty hospitals, and imaging centers all vying to take advantage of current trends. The industry has witnessed double-digit growth in the number of outpatient surgeries over the past decade. On a parallel track, diagnostic imaging has exploded, enabling earlier diagnosis and intervention. Procedures that generated significant revenue a decade ago now incur revenue loss. Former allies and partners have become competitors.

- *Increased competition for a shrinking pool of skilled labor.* There appears to be no relief in sight for the shrinking pool of skilled healthcare labor. Shortages are expected to intensify further as baby boomers retire. The U.S. Department of Labor (2004–2005) projects that registered nurses hold 2.3 million jobs, and through 2012, more jobs will be created for nurses than for any other occupation (American Hospital Association 2004). Because of a lack of nursing talent, position vacancy rates in many areas of the United States are already into double digits. The same is true for physicians. Despite increased demand, medical school admission and graduation rates have not increased since 1981.

- *Globalization of healthcare and medical tourism.* Global competition has had a profound effect on most industries, and healthcare is no different. You may have heard one of your healthcare colleagues say "all healthcare is local." This statement is based on a belief that each healthcare market is self-contained and immune to external market forces outside a limited geographic radius. In other words, what occurs in Chicago has little bearing on what happens in Atlanta. This disconnect may have existed ten years ago, but it does not today.

Nothing illustrates the changes awaiting healthcare as profoundly as the story on medical tourism aired by CBS on *60 Minutes*. Bob Simon's (2005) report described how U.S.-trained physicians and surgeons are providing world-class care in foreign countries at a fraction of the cost of the same care in the United States. The story documented the dramatic growth of medical tourism and state-of-the-art medical centers offering the most advanced medical treatments in a vacation resort environment. These facilities offer quality of care and financial incentives sufficient to induce patients to travel 12,000 miles to receive treatment. The report indicates that for a growing number of people, medical tourism has become a viable path to affordable elective and cosmetic surgery. Others see it as their best opportunity to receive expensive life-saving procedures. One of the most moving stories in the program was of a man who could not afford to pay for his heart bypass surgery. He would have incurred an estimated $100,000 out-of-pocket expense in the U.S. system. Instead, he elected to have the surgery performed overseas for $12,000.

This list of healthcare challenges is daunting, and these challenges are not going away; they are just a warm-up for tomorrow's even more complex world. With a list like this one, why are healthcare leaders surprised when there are disruptions and challenges in hospitals? Change is part of healthcare management, and senior executives must be prepared to harness that change and transform it into improved performance. Change is not something we cope with until we can get back to our regular job; leading change successfully *is* our job.

Most senior healthcare leaders know their organization's future viability and success correlate directly with the organization's ability to anticipate and respond to changes in its environment. Intellectually, leaders, managers, and staff know that those who cannot adapt and reinvent themselves are condemned to fail. Realistically, they know that maintaining the status quo is not an option. Continuing on the path of "business as usual" may delay change, but ultimately, change will catch up. Postponing change or even attempting to avoid it will make the change even more difficult to achieve.

Despite this fact, most healthcare organizations protect the status quo. They resist change even when faced with inscrutable evidence that their current care delivery processes are far from optimal, or even broken. Resistance to change has the unintended consequence of creating a widening gap between the organization's need to change and the speed at which transformational efforts occur.

HUMAN NATURE AND THE BARRIERS TO CHANGE

If change is inevitable, why do most people instinctively resist it? The simple answer is that it is against human nature. An effective change agent anticipates barriers to change and organizes efforts to surmount people's natural tendency to resist it.

To create initiatives that flow against human nature is to plan for failure. The following factors may present obstacles to achieving transformational change and must be considered when designing a new program.

- *Acceptance of the need to change is an admission of guilt.* Before change can occur, managers must acknowledge that change is needed and that their current performance and work processes are not optimal. Some perceive this acknowledgment as an admission of failure or incompetence on the manager's part. This perception may have a paralyzing effect on improvement.
- *Fear of failure and rejection trumps the desire for change.* For many individuals, the personal risk involved in change outweighs its potential rewards. Nowhere is this fear more apparent than in healthcare. Fear of failure appears to be part of healthcare's DNA. For example, clinicians are trained first to do no harm. They are taught to follow proven pathways and protocols or treatments that have been proven effective by their own experience. There is a natural bias to resist changing what works, even if there is substantial evidence supporting the use of something new. To deviate from the proven or established clinical protocols is considered acceptable only after extensive studies have demonstrated the effectiveness of a new treatment. Healthcare is a risk-averse culture. It fosters an environment that demands error-free performance and does not reward risk taking.

  Real improvements in healthcare organization processes do not come without risk. Change may incur failure. In an industry where failure is unacceptable and viewed as final or absolute, the only perceived safe and rational course of action is to maintain the status quo.

- *Comfort with the familiar leads to avoidance of change.* Fear of the unknown can stop change in its tracks. Human nature's first response to a change is to evaluate the risk and run through endless scenarios of possible negative outcomes. This type of threat assessment is a natural and organic response to a change in the environment. Regardless of how bad a current situation or process is, department managers and hospital staff are usually comfortable with it. They may acknowledge that their work processes leave much to be desired, but they fear that change to their current routines could produce an unexpected outcome that they would be unable to handle.

- *Complicated projects create the Mt. Everest syndrome.* When considering a complex task in totality, people become overwhelmed. Imagine yourself as a mountain climber facing a difficult slope. If you sit at the base of the mountain and contemplate the climb, trying to envision every step of the journey to the summit, you will become overwhelmed with the magnitude of what you must accomplish. This view has a paralyzing effect on your psyche. If you break the climb into achievable phases, your outlook changes. It becomes a series of small climbs rather than an insurmountable challenge. In a similar sense, healthcare consists of a series of complex care and work processes. When confronted with the prospect of reengineering complex work processes, managers and staff may perceive their challenges as Herculean. The size and complexity of the task may immobilize even the strongest leaders. They may perceive goals as unattainable and inadvertently diminish staff's motivation to try. As with the mountain example, breaking a complex process into several sub-processes and focusing efforts on one sub-process at a time may make the reengineering effort more manageable.

- *Discomfort with ambiguity leads to avoidance.* Most human beings are uncomfortable with even small amounts of ambiguity and uncertainty. They seek a proven map before they take the first step of a journey. Ambiguity is the root cause of many anxieties. This desire for certainty can prevent progress. Fear and protection of the status quo can masquerade as due diligence. Ambiguity can invoke a perpetual call for more data, more analysis, and examination of more alternative solutions. A guiding vision is important, but seldom does one have the luxury of knowing all the answers and details before starting a transformational initiative.

ORGANIZATIONAL BARRIERS TO CHANGE

In addition to human nature, organizational factors may present barriers to change. These barriers may prevent even the most dedicated and committed healthcare organizations from achieving desired goals. Although organizational factors that prohibit success vary from organization to organization, recurring themes tend to appear as hospitals implement new work processes. An organization can improve its probability of success by understanding and addressing these major barriers.

- *Competing priorities and lack of clear organizational focus.* Performance improvement activities require time and resources. Healthcare organizations are notorious for adding one improvement initiative on top of another. Senior leaders decide to change the current strategy and charter new task-forces and work teams without disbanding the former ones. At some point, the organization passes the tipping point and change grinds to a halt. Managers are frustrated because they spend all their time in meetings and have minimal time to implement needed improvements. Focus remains on the urgent rather than on strategically important issues. These symptoms signal that the hospital has no systematic and strategic way of assigning priorities or ensuring that the resources for change are sufficient and focused on improving important core processes.

Perpetual priority shifts cause managers and staff to develop a resistance to the directions of leadership. Even well-meaning managers may be slow to act because of confusion about organizational priorities. Other managers may adopt a strategy of keeping a low profile because they know the next "daily crisis" will postpone the need for them to act today. In the *Harvard Business Review* article "Change Through Persuasion," Garvin and Roberto (2005) claim that "Where leaders repeatedly proclaimed a state of crisis but made few substantive changes, employees became jaded. They developed a bunker mentality. The wisest course of action is to ignore new initiatives."

- *Misaligned incentives.* Changes in work processes and department interactions may create misaligned incentives— formal or informal rewards that put individual interests at odds with organizational interests. For example, managers may resist using staff more efficiently if they perceive that doing so will reduce their number of direct reports and thus diminish their standing in the organization. Likewise, a laboratory manager may seek to optimize personal performance by batching lab results to improve the efficiency and costs of producing a diagnostic result. Batching would allow the lab director to minimize reagent utilization, labor, and other costs per test result, thus achieving financial targets. However, excessive batching of test results typically delays the release of patient data, thereby hindering the physician's ability to write timely discharge orders for patients. Although the lab is meeting its cost goals per test result, the hospital is incurring excess labor costs and losing revenue while it cares for patients who should have been discharged. This project-by-project approach often creates misaligned incentives that cost the hospital millions in lost revenue and expenses related to poor patient flow. When senior leaders delegate project selection and performance improvement down to the manager level, the result is a project-by-project approach that focuses efforts on insignificant tactical issues and proliferates misaligned incentives.

- *Benchmarking's potential to paralyze.* The concept of comparative data swept across healthcare approximately 20 years ago. Today, data comparison, or benchmarking, is a multibillion-dollar industry. On the surface, the concept of benchmarking is straightforward and logical. You compare your performance to others, which helps you to find opportunity for improvement. Unfortunately, benchmarking has paralyzed more healthcare organizations than it has helped. Healthcare institutions spend excessive amounts of time, money, and human capital arguing about the accuracy of data instead of using this time to implement needed changes. Benchmarking data are valuable, but the way most healthcare organizations use these data slows progress and creates barriers to action. Benchmarking can be a useful exercise if it incites a hospital to act, but not if it causes further delays and protects the status quo.

- *Ineffectiveness of external standards and best practices.* As with benchmarking, organizations have expended tremendous resources to identify healthcare best practices. Some of the industry's greatest minds have focused on isolating the clinical practices of top-performing hospitals and departments across the country. This research is based on a prevalent belief that if organizations can identify the nation's top-performing emergency room, surgery department, or nursing model, they can emulate its care processes in their facilities.

    Unfortunately, direct import of best practices seldom produces success or lasting change. The concept of best practices assumes that each emergency department is operating in the same environment and is experiencing the same constraints and bottlenecks. Healthcare is too complex for hospitals to be identical. Therefore, the premise on which the best practice model is based is inherently flawed.

The best practice approach also assumes that best practices can be imposed on staff without cultivating belief in the proposed change. Consultants often issue reports containing manifold well-vetted best practices only to have staff reject them. The hospital staff even may agree to implement the proposed changes in a half-hearted fashion to prove the consultant's recommendations were wrong. Even when the recommendations show promise, gains dissipate once the consultant leaves and hospital staff members drift back to their old work patterns. Without taking the necessary steps to foster belief in the change and to hardwire improved work processes, lasting results will not ensue.

Identifying best practices is a valuable step in designing new work processes, and much can be learned from examining the practices of other providers, but senior leaders must recognize that every hospital has its own complex interconnected work processes and culture.

- *Overreliance on monitoring systems.* Hospitals are striving to catch up with other industries in their use of information technology. Senior leaders are staking their careers and futures on multimillion-dollar investments in monitoring systems. The prevalent belief in healthcare is that if we only had a way to monitor the problem, we would know what to do and the problem would correct itself. Research indicates that hospitals that see monitoring systems as the prime solution to driving improvement are headed for disappointment.

- *Inadequate accountability.* Hospitals have moved toward a more collaborative environment in the past few decades, using multidisciplinary teams, creating task forces, and developing a number of shared governance structures. This team approach provides staff with the opportunity to express viewpoints on critical issues. Unfortunately, these collaborative efforts have not produced the level of change and transformation their creators had anticipated. Objective observation of many of these teams in action reveals that they have degenerated into gripe sessions, social clubs, and monitoring organizations. Teams spend a minimal amount of time, if any, implementing and pursuing solutions. They spend most of their time discussing issues or monitoring clinical metrics rather than singling out one issue to improve before the next meeting. Senior leaders frequently express concern about this lack of accountability for producing tangible results. When everyone is responsible for a result, nobody appears responsible. In many cases, these multidisciplinary teams mask inaction and protect the status quo.

A CALL TO ACTION

The quickening pace of change has heightened the importance of leading transformational efforts and made such leadership a highly valued executive core competency. The current healthcare environment demands that senior executives develop specific leadership skills to guide their organization through transformational efforts and coach managers in the methods of change.

Change is unavoidable. The logical response is to develop a deliberate strategy for embracing it and harnessing its energy. The following chapters discuss how senior leaders can embrace their role as change leaders and develop accountability for change, create an environment conducive to change, and link strategies to quality outcomes.

REFERENCES

American Hospital Association. 2004. *Stat: Tackling Today's Challenges, Addressing Workforce Shortages.* Annual Meeting Paper, July 28.

Anderson, G. 2000. "Quality and Innovation: Issues, Strategies, and Implications for Policy." Commonwealth Fund International Symposium on Health Care Policy, Washington, DC, October 11–13. [Online information; retrieved 6/20/08.] http://content.healthaffairs.org/cgi/content/full/20/3/219#T5.

Baker, S. L. 2007. "U.S. National Health Spending, 2005." [Online information; retrieved 6/27/08.] http://hadm.sph.sc.edu/COURSES/Econ/Classes/nhe00.

Fisch, K., and S. McLeod. 2007. "Did You Know 2.0." Washington, DC: U.S. Chamber of Commerce, June 22. [Online information; retrieved 6/27/08.] www.youtube.com/watch?v=pMcfrLYDm2U.

Garvin, D., and M. Roberto. 2005. "Change Through Persuasion." *Harvard Business Review* 83 (2): 104.

Simon, B. 2005. "Vacation, Adventure and Surgery." *60 Minutes*, CBS, September 4.

U.S. Census Bureau. 2000. "Census 2000." [Online information; retrieved 6/20/08.] www.census.gov.

U.S. Department of Labor, Bureau of Labor Statistics, Office of Occupational Statistics and Employment Projections. 2004–2005. "Occupational Outlook Handbook." [Online information; retrieved 12/19/07.] www.bls.gov/oco/home.htm.

World Health Organization. 2000. *The World Health Report 2000—Health Systems: Improving Performance*. Geneva, Switzerland, June 1.

CHAPTER 2

The Characteristics
of Success

To improve is to change. To be perfect is to change often.
—Winston Churchill (1874–1965)

ALL HOSPITALS HAVE strategic plans, budgets, and hopes for success and improved performance. Unfortunately, good intentions do not necessarily yield good results. What separates high-performing or "quantum improver" organizations from "nonstarter" organizations that struggle with success? Do they have attributes or characteristics that can be isolated and reproduced? How does senior leadership foster these characteristics?

Research originally published by the American College of Healthcare Executives under the title "'Good to Great' in Healthcare: How Some Organizations Are Elevating Their Performance" (Pieper 2004) began to answer these questions. We continued the task by studying the work of hundreds of organizations across the country. We looked at certain financial indicators to segment these organizations into quartiles, designating the highest-performing hospitals as quantum improvers and the lowest-performing hospitals as nonstarters. Through this research, we discovered that quantum improver organizations possess certain characteristics and attributes. Their attitudes about performance improvement efforts as well as their strategies for benchmarking, goal setting, and using technology work together to help them succeed.

ATTITUDES AND ROLES

There are distinct differences in how leaders and managers in quantum improver and nonstarter organizations see their roles in the organization. Leaders and managers in quantum improver organizations exude a passion for challenging the status quo and improving work processes. Their senior leaders consider performance improvement as part of their job descriptions and incorporate this philosophy into the daily fabric of their work. Mark Tolosky (2004), CEO of Baystate Health in Springfield, Massachusetts—one of the quantum improver organizations we identified—remarked that the organization's success came not from the effectiveness of its strategic planning process but rather from the strength of leadership's cultural bias at all levels of the organization. He emphasized that managers were passionate about achieving excellence in all dimensions of their performance and that this characteristic accounted more for the organization's continued success than did the words of its strategic plan.

In contrast, leaders and managers in nonstarter organizations see performance improvement and change management as an episodic and extracurricular activity rather than as an ongoing process, and they tolerate such activity until they can get back to their regular jobs. A prevalent attitude among nonstarter leaders and managers is that their primary job is to maintain existing operations.

Our research indicated that senior leaders of quantum improver organizations understand the need to create an environment of change in which managers are recognized and rewarded for taking calculated risks. Failure in these organizations is a natural part of a learning process that leads to ultimate progress and success. In contrast, managers of nonstarter organizations see even the smallest failure as a final judgment with personal repercussions—something they must avoid.

Table 2.1 lists some opposing characteristics of quantum improver and nonstarter managers.

Table 2.1 Quantum Improver Versus Nonstarter Manager Attributes

Quantum Improver Managers	Nonstarter Managers
Appear confident	Appear afraid of change
Handle ambiguity well	Focus on unknown; allow naysayers and gaps in data to delay action
Actively seek to change the status quo	Find comfort in the status quo
Question traditions and customs; are inquisitive	Seek to protect customs and traditions
Show bias toward action over analysis	See uncertainty as a reason to delay action; enjoy analysis
Persist and do not see failure as a final judgment	See failure as a final judgment
Are persuasive	Are uncomfortable expressing ideas and rationales
Are motivated by praise and recognition	May shun attention
Approach risk management in a balanced manner	Appear to treat all risk the same
Reduce complex issues to manageable components	Are overwhelmed by the complexity of proposed changes

KNOWLEDGE APPLICATION

Our research correlated organizational performance with the presence of quality acceleration methods, such as Lean-Six Sigma and the Toyota Production System. We hypothesized that organizations that had invested in quality acceleration methods would have superior performance. However, our analysis revealed this hypothesis as false. There was no statistical correlation between the presence and absence of quality acceleration methods. In fact, quantum improver organizations ranked quality acceleration methods 30 percent lower than other methods as drivers of change. In other words, the use of quality acceleration methods alone was not a predictor of superior performance.

Interesting patterns emerged from the research that built on this observation. We discovered that nonstarter organizations believe that training is essential to driving improvement through quality acceleration methods. For nonstarters, training is a goal that culminates with the placement of good-looking binders on every manager's bookshelf. Quantum improvers recognize that training alone does not ensure success but that it is the beginning of a longer process of knowledge acquisition. Quantum improvers realize that when training is complete, the real work begins. They have a plan for the systematic application of the new knowledge and tools they have acquired. Quantum improver organizations apply this training by insisting that managers demonstrate use of these new tools and methods at monthly performance reviews.

Consider this example. Quantum improver organization Floyd Regional Medical Center in Rome, Georgia, was at least one generation behind in the sophistication of its quality methods, yet the organization achieved top-quartile performance. The differentiator, according to Sonny Rigas (2004), chief operating officer, was the disciplined adherence to an accountability system characterized by rapid goal setting and action planning, and a monthly results check-in process in which senior leaders and managers held each other accountable for completing action plans. These meetings were not punitive; they were coaching sessions that occurred frequently if progress was at risk. Systematic follow-up tracked employees' integration of new tools into their daily work.

BENCHMARKING

We were startled to discover that the traditional approach to benchmarking can slow progress and prevent change. Quantum improvers have escaped this trap and are applying new benchmarking strategies. First, senior executives of quantum improvers realize that the singular purpose for benchmarking is to identify opportunity and move people to action. Second, they understand that speed to action is the most important variable. When they benchmark, quantum improvers look at a large comparative sample. Typically, they use an aggressive broad peer group of 500 or more hospitals rather than a narrow group of 5 hospitals. They have learned how to avoid arguing about the data, how to avoid shopping for new peer groups, and how to break the endless cycle of analysis.

In all the quantum improver organizations interviewed, no more than 30 days elapsed from the start of the benchmarking process until senior leaders finalized goals with managers. To keep the process brief, these senior leaders began by acknowledging that all benchmarking data are flawed. Instead of allowing a debilitating debate on the accuracy of benchmarking data, they acknowledged at the front end of the process that there is no such thing as a perfect peer group. Most managers cannot justify the claim that data are more than 10 to 15 percent inaccurate. Senior leaders asserted that if no one could argue that the data were 50 percent bad, their goal would be to close half the gap between their organization and the benchmarked organizations. They then requested immediate turnaround of action plans, which ended the discussion about data validity and moved managers rapidly into implementation.

Consider this example. Floyd Regional Medical Center recognized that the traditional approach to benchmarking was delaying the implementation of manager action plans. Therefore, rather than argue about the validity of the comparison group, senior leaders set manager goals at the 65th percentile and set a 30-day deadline for manager action plans.

Contrast Floyd Regional Medical Center's approach with that of a large nonstarter hospital in Detroit, which earned its bottom-quartile designation not because of a lack of manager expertise or the availability of credible data but because of a culture that accepted manager denial and protected the status quo. Rather than follow quantum improvers' speedy approach, this organization debated for 11 months about the appropriateness of the selected peer group, the validity of the data provided to the comparative benchmarking firm, and the relevance of other hospitals' best practices.

GOAL SETTING

Quantum improvers separate goal setting from the identification of solutions, whereas nonstarters tend to set goals only after they have identified a total solution. For example, let's say a senior adminis-trator discusses benchmarks with managers suggesting an opportu-nity. Reasonable managers would ask whether they could call their counterparts at the benchmarked hospitals. If the senior adminis-trator has not established firm performance improvement goals (characteristic of nonstarter organizations), the purpose of these calls tends to be to judge the practices of the peer hospital rather than to uncover solutions. By the end of the call, the manager has a notepad of reasons why the practices of the peer hospital will not work in his or her department. This exercise in "best practices" has become an exercise in defending the status quo.

On the other hand, if the senior administrator has set firm goals with the manager, only the best strategy to achieve the desired result remains in question. By establishing firm goals first, quantum improver organizations change the purpose of the call from evaluating the goal to uncovering potential solutions for improving performance. Because the status quo is not an option, the manager's intent is to determine how to make these strategies work in his or her department. The manager exerts mental energy figuring out how to adapt and modify the work processes of a peer hospital to work in the manager's organization.

STRATEGY DEPLOYMENT

Some form of performance improvement initiative is underway in all healthcare organizations. However, a quantum improver organization and a nonstarter organization respond differently when asked to describe their performance improvement initiatives. Nonstarters tend to provide a long list of projects with limited connections to larger operating strategies of the hospital. Nonstarters seem to select their performance improvement projects in an ad hoc manner or in response to a series of imagined crises and knee-jerk requests. In contrast, quantum improver organizations provide a clear and concise statement covering three or four key strategies. They understand the importance of linking their performance improvement efforts to their major strategic operational goals and have identified their core processes clearly. They know which goals warrant the attention of senior leaders and are integral to the organization's success. Quantum improver organizations understand that strategy and quality improvement prioritization are inseparable. They know their organizations have a finite capacity to change at any given moment and prefer to focus the organization's resources on improving one or two larger core operating processes.

Quantum improvers understand the importance of focus on interdepartmental, cross-functional core processes in driving change. Although performance improvement happens one project at a time, when performance improvement lacks a grand design and unified effort to improve a major core process, improvement efforts in one area may hinder improvement in another.

TECHNOLOGY APPLICATION

Quantum improver organizations view and deploy technology differently than nonstarter organizations do. One would assume that quantum improvers have made significant investments in sophisticated information technology (IT) solutions and have harnessed data to achieve stellar performance. In reality, we observed no differences between the two types of healthcare organizations' IT spending.

Explanation for this lack of difference lies in how healthcare organizations view technology and data. Many of the nonstarters have made significant investments in elaborate IT systems and are collecting impressive amounts of data. However, they approach their efforts more as an academic exercise than as an integrated decision. They give minimal forethought to how to integrate the data into the operations of the hospital or specific departments, and there is no expectation in the organization's culture that a manager take action when confronted with data indicating a deviation from targets and goals.

In contrast, quantum improvers do not collect data for the sake of monitoring alone. Many of the quantum improver organizations we interviewed went the extra step to ensure that a result that deviated from an expected value triggered a formal response process. Quantum improvers know that an unexpected result or a deviation from the plan is a sign that their work processes may be flawed and that they must investigate and correct it to yield the desired result.

For quantum improvers, work process redesign is the primary consideration when reviewing the application of technology. They first discuss how they will transform their work processes and the role technology can play in this redesign. These organizations understand that they make true gains in performance only when technology facilitates a tangible change in work processes. They establish clear expectations that investments in technology will transform work processes and yield tangible gains in capacity, increased productivity, and other forms of cost recovery.

LESSONS LEARNED ACROSS INDUSTRIES

These good-to-best conclusions are similar to those of other studies on transformational initiatives. One notable work is that of John Kotter, a Harvard University professor who is widely regarded as the world's foremost authority on leadership and change. Over the past 20 years, Kotter has studied the art of leading change across a diversity of companies and industries and published more than 16 books on the subject of change management. One of his most notable works centered on a list of eight primary reasons why change initiatives fail (Kotter 1995):

- Error 1: Not establishing a great enough sense of urgency
- Error 2: Not creating a powerful enough guiding coalition
- Error 3: Lacking a vision
- Error 4: Undercommunicating the vision by a factor of ten
- Error 5: Not removing obstacles to the new vision
- Error 6: Not planning and creating short-term wins systematically
- Error 7: Declaring victory too soon
- Error 8: Not anchoring changes in the corporation's culture

Our research indicated that there are distinct organizational attributes that correlate with success. Harold Sirkin conducted a study of 225 organizations to isolate other dimensions influencing the success of change initiatives and identified many of the same attributes (Sirkin, Keenan, and Jackson 2005). The conclusions from Sirkin's research indicated there are tangible, measurable characteristics related to how transformational efforts are organized. He developed a correlation between the following four organizational attributes (called the DICE score) that successfully predicted the future success of transformational initiatives:

- Duration
- Integrity

- Commitment of senior leaders and staff
- Effort

HOW TO BECOME A QUANTUM IMPROVER ORGANIZATION

We have discussed why to improve and what to improve, but the most crucial aspect of our work entails how to improve. How can senior leaders achieve the characteristics associated with quantum improver organizations? How can they make performance improvement part of the organization's daily work? How can they create realistic goals and empower staff to achieve them? How can they move from ideas to action?

Senior executives can create a dynamic vision, but there is no realization without execution. Execution requires senior leaders to link their vision to organizational performance, create an environment of change, and design a structure of accountability. Senior leaders also must create a unifying structure that concentrates resources on achieving specific results.

For organizations to achieve the "how" of performance improvement at the quantum improver level, senior leaders must embrace the four following nondelegable roles (Caldwell 2008).

- *Design and implement an accountability system.* Accountability systems are methods of reporting that make progress or its absence instantly visible. These systems involve regular, consistent, and organization-wide communication about performance improvement projects occurring within the organization and establish responsibility and accountability for completing those projects. They allow organizations to prioritize and interrelate performance improvement initiatives to ensure progress.
- *Link strategy to quality.* Senior leaders must identify mega core processes integral to the overall performance of the organization. These work processes define what makes a hospital a hospital

or a clinic a clinic. Without clearly defining these large processes, senior leaders will have difficulty gaining significant traction in their quality and performance improvement initiatives. Once senior leaders have identified them, they can create focus by selecting projects that improve these large core processes and thus produce strategic results for the organization. Failure to do so results in an unfocused, project-by-project approach that produces marginal results.

- *Create an environment for change.* Leaders must establish and communicate a strategic vision, promote change, support failure, and encourage speed to action.
- *Use advanced quality methods effectively.* As previously mentioned, advanced quality methods alone are not predictors of success. However, when an organization uses advanced quality methods effectively, it can accelerate gains by identifying critical processes that require improvement and creating a disciplined, systematic approach to implementation. Knowing when and how to use the variety of advanced quality methods is paramount to achieving success. See Figure 2.1.

Figure 2.1 Four Elements of Quantum Improvers' Success

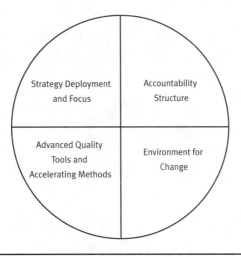

The following four chapters take a closer look at these four efforts and provide specific examples of how organizations can engage in these efforts and achieve transformational change.

REFERENCES

Caldwell, C. 2008. "Aggressively Improve Costs and Throughput Using Lean Six Sigma." Seminar presented by American College of Healthcare Executives, Keystone, CO, January 30–31.

Kotter, J. 1995. "Leading Change: Why Transformational Efforts Fail." *Harvard Business Review* 73 (2): 59–67.

Pieper, S. 2004. "'Good to Great' in Healthcare: How Some Organizations Are Elevating Their Performance." *Healthcare Executive* 19 (3): 20–26.

Rigas, S. (COO, Floyd Regional Medical Center), in discussion with the authors, March 17, 2004.

Sirkin, H., P. Keenan, and A. Jackson. 2005. "The Hard Side of Change Management." *Harvard Business Review* 83 (10): 108–18.

Tolosky, M. (president and CEO, Baystate Health), in discussion with the authors, March 4, 2004.

CHAPTER 3

Organizing for Accountability

Change is the law of life and those who look only to the past or present are certain to miss the future.

—John F. Kennedy

THE WORD *ACCOUNTABILITY* conjures up notions of judgment and consequence. These ideas are inaccurate. Pieper's (2004) healthcare research identified that quantum improver organizations have a systematic, structural view of accountability and deliberately design their work to ensure that they progress. A strong accountability system can help senior leaders focus their attention on achieving specific, strategic results while creating regular opportunities for collaboration and information sharing across departmental boundaries. Such a system makes performance improvement routine rather than episodic.

An accountability system comprises reports, meetings, and other tools that make an organization's progress instantly visible. Critical attributes of a strong accountability system include the frequency of check-ins, involvement of senior leaders, transparency of progress, and the structural and cultural elements of the environment of change (see Chapter 6).

THE EVOLUTION OF ACCOUNTABILITY SYSTEMS

During the 1980s and 1990s, large, complex manufacturers such as General Motors and General Electric (GE) struggled with accountability and their ability to compete and respond rapidly to changing market conditions and opportunities. Multiple layers of bureaucracy and organizational hierarchy prevented these organizations from realizing their full potential. In response, organizations began developing uniform methods of driving change.

One example is the GE Workout structure, which became the main structure for enhancing accountability and the speed of change (Ulrich 2002). The GE Workout structure was a summit (multiday event) dedicated to improving a specific aspect of a work process. Senior leaders assembled an ad hoc team to participate in the Workout, consisting of the managers who owned the process to be improved and those with authority to grant necessary approvals or technical expertise to guide the process.

Once assembled, the team held an intense meeting designed to achieve action and rapid results. The team continued to meet over a two- to three-day period until the group identified opportunities for improvement, developed plans, assigned accountability to specific team members, and set out to implement the changes. Team members suspended their regular duties to focus on implementing solutions. The goals for the Workout structure were to:

- realize tangible gains within a short time;
- achieve speed to action with an emphasis on implementation;
- reduce bureaucratic barriers that hinder decision making and approvals;
- expose and overcome misalignment of incentives;
- generate ideas at every level of the organization;
- increase the visibility of results; and
- improve accountability at every level of the organization.

The industrial model for the Workout was well suited for manufacturing and business processes. In theory, it seems applicable to the healthcare environment, but it has proven to be impractical in the hospital environment for the following reasons.

- Healthcare providers seldom have the luxury of removing themselves from the normal work environment for multiple days at a time to work on a specific problem.
- Redesign and testing of healthcare processes are difficult to complete in the two- to three-day period of the typical Workout.
- The Workout method did not incorporate mechanisms that build healthcare practitioners' belief in change.
- The Workout method focused on a set of projects instead of promoting an ongoing performance improvement process.

Despite these shortcomings, the Workout's structure contains many elements of a strong accountability system. It offers senior leadership-driven, focused time frames for achieving strategic performance improvement. It is interdepartmental and helps organizations realize short-term wins.

THE 100-DAY QUALITY WORKOUT FOR HEALTHCARE

Several years ago, we took the positive attributes of all accountability systems and amalgamated the suitable components into an effective process. We created a process tailored for the healthcare workplace, called the "100-Day Quality Workout." Over the past five years, we have tested the 100-Day Quality Workout and have found that it improved a hospital's ability to execute and achieve meaningful gains in operating and clinical performance. This method proved to be most reliable and efficient in organizing healthcare professionals for change and creating a culture of action and accountability.

We did not design the 100-Day Quality Workout to be a one-time event but rather a uniform system of conducting the business of performance improvement. It provides a set of principles and methods that allow for differences in culture, as well as a comprehensive system for managing every aspect of a hospital's performance improvement initiatives and deployment of quality resources. The goals of the 100-Day Quality Workout include:

- making progress or its absence instantly visible throughout the organization;
- focusing the entire organization on achieving improvements in major core processes;
- establishing a common way of doing business that spans the organization;
- creating a perpetual environment of improvement;
- eliminating unnecessary meetings and nonproductive teams and committees;
- improving accountability at every level in the organization by providing transparency for the accurate assessment of progress;
- accelerating the creation of meaningful benchmarks and goals while improving employee acceptance of targets; and
- overcoming the natural fears that most managers have of change and creating a bias for action.

CREATING AN URGENCY FOR CHANGE

Creating a sense of urgency is a vital component to driving change, and the ideal accountability system moves people from planning to action. Long intervals between reviews of performance improvement initiatives, such as six months or a year, can diminish the sense of urgency and increase the probability that an organization's results will slip. In these cases, too much time elapses before performance improvement activities surface to the top of a manager's priority list (Kotter 1995).

For this reason, we suggest organizing performance improvement into three 100-day cycles with a 20-day assessment break between each cycle. We also suggest a monthly check-in during each 100-day implementation period. The rationale for selecting 100 days follows.

- Hundred-day cycles allow sufficient time for teams to implement meaningful improvements that move initiatives forward. Shorter time cycles do not provide for a critical mass of changes within sub-processes to make progress on strategic goals.
- Hundred-day cycles are short enough to create a true sense of urgency in most organizations.
- Hundred-day cycles prevent the performance improvement process from linking to the budget cycle.

CREATING DEDICATED TIME FOR ACTION AND PLANNING

One of the key elements in the 100-Day Quality Workout is time dedicated to implementation. Such allocation maintains the focus on action and moving forward. By the end of the 20-day break between cycles, all analysis and planning for the current cycle should be completed and action should be initiated. If new ideas emerge, they are to be captured and included in the next 100-day improvement cycle. Strict cycles break the bad habit of perpetually restarting efforts as new ideas and strategies are interjected into the performance improvement process.

Consider this example. A 400-bed hospital system in Arizona established a goal of eliminating $5 million in quality waste during its first 100-Day Quality Workout. After training in quality waste recovery, managers identified more than $6.5 million in quality waste during the first 20 days of planning. At the 30-day mark, managers still were generating new ideas and demanding more tools and training. Although they were successful at identifying opportunities, few managers had implemented the changes they had identified. During a session with the executive team, we asked team members why they wanted to generate more ideas and provide more training when their staff already had more ideas than it could implement during the next 100 days. The executive team agreed and encouraged managers to stop adding more items to their current 100-day action plans and to focus their attention on implementing the items already in their plans. When managers came up with another big idea, the executive team told them to put it in the next 100-Day Quality Workout planning folder. These steps kept the organization focused on implementation. The net result of this focus produced tangible financial gains approaching $7 million.

Figure 3.1 illustrates the structure of the 100-Day Quality Workout accountability system. Dedicating specific time to implementation ensures that a minimum of 75 percent of the time is spent in these cycles. This figure is opposite that of nonstarter organizations, which we found spent greater than 75 percent of their time in the planning mode.

SEPARATING PERFORMANCE IMPROVEMENT FROM THE BUDGET

Organizations often design accountability systems and reviews of performance improvement initiatives to coincide with their financial cycles and accounting reporting periods, typically every 90 days.

Figure 3.1 100-Day Workout Productivity Cycle

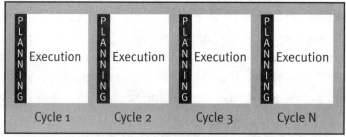

Allocate 25% to Planning and 75% to Execution

Synchronizing an accountability system with the budget review cycle is a problem because managers fear the immediate inclusion of changes in their budgets. This fear thwarts positive energy. Managers must believe they can test and validate changes before they become a permanent part of the operating budget. Without a safe environment to propose, test, and validate performance improvement ideas, managers may withhold creative ideas.

Consider this example. A 100-bed rehabilitation hospital in the Chicago area was making excellent progress eliminating waste from the organization. Progress came to an abrupt halt when the chief financial officer insisted on integrating the budget review process with managers' efforts to eliminate quality waste. Managers feared that any idea they communicated would result in an immediate reduction in their budgets, whether or not their ideas produced sustainable savings. Previously, managers felt safe proposing changes and knew they would have an opportunity to test their ideas and hardwire the changes in work processes before their budgets were adjusted. The chief financial officer's desire to couple the performance improvement efforts with the annual budget process drove all efforts underground until after the budget process was complete. This suppression created a significant loss of momentum and severed the managers' trust.

In contrast, Floyd Regional Medical Center maintained a reasonable separation between the budget process and the 100-Day Quality Workout process, choosing to incorporate manager innovations into the budget only after managers expressed confidence that their efforts were sustainable. This organization's chief financial officer was rewarded with more than $6 million in validated quality cost recovery in the first 100 days (Stuenkel and Caldwell 2008).

FOUR KEY ROLES IN THE 100-DAY QUALITY WORKOUT

To manage the 100-Day Quality Workout successfully, the chief executive officer must designate four key roles:

- Executive champion
- Workout coordinator
- Finance liaison
- Communication coordinator

Executive Champion

The chief executive officer must designate an individual from the senior leadership team to serve as an executive champion and spokesperson for each 100-Day Quality Workout. The executive champion's primary role is to serve as the central face and voice of the senior leadership team during implementation. The executive champion must have full support of the senior leadership team to ensure that the process maintains momentum. The executive champion's main responsibilities include:

- gaining senior team consensus on the focus of the 100-Day Quality Workout;
- fine-tuning the 100-Day Quality Workout to the specific culture of the organization;
- identifying and assigning key resources;
- selecting individuals to fill key roles;
- facilitating data requests;
- guiding the development and implementation of the communication plan;
- overseeing meetings, calendars, and events;
- working with the finance department in the validation of results; and
- aggregating and reporting cumulative results.

When selecting the executive champion, consider individuals who have the following attributes:

- Presence on the senior leadership team

- Positional authority to access and coordinate the organization's resources
- Deep understanding of the organization's strategy and priorities
- Desire to serve and passion for transformational efforts
- Ability to dedicate four to eight hours per month to performance improvement

Workout Coordinator

Workout coordinators assist the executive champion in managing the logistics of the 100-Day Quality Workout. They support managers in understanding the 100-Day Quality Workout process and serve as an access point to tools and resources. In addition, workout coordinators support executive champions by serving as eyes and ears during each cycle of the Workout. They frequently interact with managers charged with making changes to their work processes. A capable workout coordinator can use this opportunity to provide the executive champion with a sense of how communications are received, which managers are achieving their assigned goals, and which need coaching, as well as track the overall progress of the organization. The workout coordinator's responsibilities include:

- supporting timely development of 100-day action plans;
- communicating the status of 100-day action plans to key executives;
- identifying potential successes and challenges;
- distributing performance goals and targets;
- collecting and auditing 100-day action plans;
- coordinating calendar and meetings; and
- providing limited idea-generation support to stimulate discussions.

Recommend resources for the workout coordinator include:

- Healthcare Advisory Board best practice reports;
- medical publications/journals/reprints;
- medical professional associations/standards and best practices; and
- quality improvement tools, such as Six Sigma and rapid cycle testing.

We recommend that management designate, mentor, and apprentice one to four employees, depending on the size of the organization, in the 100-Day Quality Workout methodology to serve as workout coordinators.

Formal training as a quality professional is not necessary to be effective in implementing the 100-Day Quality Workout methodology. We recommend that senior leadership identify individuals who:

- have a desire to serve;
- show aptitude for project management;
- demonstrate the ability to break complex projects into simpler tasks;
- have a strong track record for moving projects to completion;
- have excellent organizational skills;
- are respected by other employees in the hospital;
- have solid communication skills; and
- are able to commit two to three days per month to organizing activities.

Finance Liaison

The finance liaison creates a relationship between clinical managers who know care processes and the individuals who understand cost accounting and have the financial training to quantify the impact of proposed changes. Designation of a finance liaison is an important step toward ensuring that the organization receives a tangible return on its performance improvement efforts. The finance liaison role has the following responsibilities.

- Assisting managers in the quantification of savings derived from implementing changes in work processes, which includes reviewing results posted by the manager to ensure the integrity of the methodology used to quantify savings. The finance liaison ensures that gains are tangible and will produce measurable savings and assists in the development of a uniform standard of gain measurement that reduces variation from department to department.
- Providing managers with a conduit to the necessary financial data required for the 100-Day Quality Workout and analyzing departmental performance.
- Tracking the changes made by managers for the purpose of integrating tangible gains into the organization's operating budget.
- Maintaining reporting integrity by counting only hard cost savings and preventing soft costs from entering the calculations. (We recommend that soft costs not be counted in return on investment calculations.)

We recommend that senior leadership identify individuals who:

- are approachable by clinical managers;
- possess intimate knowledge of the hospital's cost centers and account systems;
- have access to the hospital's accounting and financial systems;
- are able to dedicate one to two days per month to supporting performance improvement activities; and
- have a desire to serve.

Communication Coordinator

The communication coordinator's main role is to help the executive champion communicate with the organization effectively. The communication coordinator's key roles and responsibilities include:

- assisting the executive champion in creating an effective message, which may include creating a campaign name or theme that supports the organization's goals;
- creating an effective communication plan that harnesses all the communication channels in the organization, such as newsletters, e-mail, and the hospital's intranet;
- communicating the steps in the 100-Day Quality Workout process;
- attending the monthly check-ins, capturing information from managers' reports, and selecting stories for newsletters and other communications; and
- assisting the executive champion in planning the celebration that occurs at the end of a 100-day cycle by supplying the executive champion with creative ideas that make the celebration and awards fun and exciting.

We recommend that senior leadership identify individuals who have the following attributes:

- Familiarity with the organization's brand message and employee communications
- Positional authority to direct the placement of stories highlighting the organization's performance improvement efforts
- Understanding of the organization's key strategies for improving operations
- Ability to attend the two- to three-hour monthly check-ins and the time and ability to translate the reports into success stories

STRUCTURE OF THE 100-DAY QUALITY WORKOUT

We suggest the following structure for the 100-Day Quality Workout:

- Kickoff (all-day event to start the process)
- 30-day check-in (two-hour meeting)
- 60-day check-in (two-hour meeting)
- 90-day check-in (two-hour meeting)
- Summation/next kickoff (all-day event that starts the next 100-day cycle)

The Kickoff

The kickoff is an all-day event and requires the participation of the work process owners involved in the strategic focus of the 100-Day Quality Workout. Every kickoff has the following five critical objectives.

- *Name a strategic process focus.* Senior leadership must establish a clear statement about the purpose and goals of the 100-Day Quality Workout. The executive champion must present a strong case for change and create a sense of urgency among participating managers.
- *Establish a challenge.* Every kickoff should contain an expectation of what each individual and team are to accomplish in the next 100 days. The challenge can take the form of implementations of successful changes, accomplishments of key tasks, or recovery of tangible costs. Our research shows that quantum improvers place more importance on activity-based targets than on financial goals. No manager should leave the kickoff unclear about what executive leadership expects him or her to accomplish by the end of the 100-Day Quality Workout cycle.
- *Incorporate continuing education.* Experience shows that the best approach to incorporating continuing education is to expose managers to the tools they will use in the following 100 days to accomplish the challenge issued by senior leadership. Providing managers with new methods and tools at the start of each cycle accomplishes several vital tasks. It keeps the staff growing in its

capabilities, and it prevents the program from becoming stale and boring. Most important, it provides training in a learning environment that promotes the integration of new methods into the organization's daily work. Managers benefit more from focusing on a set of tools they can master than from ten days of theory in a classroom setting. The key to success is keeping the educational session to no more than two hours. New tools should be limited to ones managers will use during the 100-Day Quality Workout. Training on tools that managers will not use during the 100-Day Quality Workout is a distraction from the Workout's focus.

- *Create a practicum or exercise.* A practicum moves participants from theory to practical application. It consists of exercises that test the participating managers' understanding of the tools presented during the educational session and ability to apply them. The practicum should create a safe learning experience where managers can admit whether they need additional instruction or clarification.

- *Create action plans by the end of the kickoff.* A kickoff should not end before every participant has initiated his or her action plan. Never hold a kickoff meeting without the clear expectation that action plans will be required by the end of the day. Planning may not be complete by the end of a kickoff, but every participant's plan must list at least two action items. Research shows that ending a kickoff without initiation of action plans leads to delayed results or Workout failure.

30-, 60-, and 90-Day Check-Ins

Monthly check-ins drive accountability. Check-ins should be structured as two- to three-hour meetings in which the executive champion or executive team leaders ask team members to provide updates on their progress. Check-ins should be kept as concise and brief as possible but should be long enough to assess progress and teach.

All participants in the 100-Day Quality Workout should attend the monthly check-ins. The meeting should be a forum in which everyone can participate and ask questions.

Set Regular Meeting Dates

Hospitals should set regular dates for the check-ins versus scheduling them on an ad hoc basis. Participants will understand that check-ins occur regardless of their personal schedules, and a regularly scheduled check-in time maintains a sense of urgency and prevents slippage. The process must continue with or without the individual. Organizations that wait for the synchronization of individual calendars suffer from poor results. Participating managers know that once a month there will be a public discussion of progress, and their progress will be visible to the organization.

Executive Leadership Drives the Meeting

Executive champions initiate every meeting with a three- to five-minute inspirational overview, reiterating and reinforcing the goals and objectives for the current 100-Day Quality Workout. This repetition drives the right message into every level of the organization, counters emerging objections, and corrects misperceptions.

Executive team leaders should facilitate the reports of their respective areas or teams. These leaders should be called to the front of the room to preside before their teams actually give their reports. The physical presence of the executive leader in front of the team reinforces his or her commitment and accountability. Research has shown that results diminish when senior leaders are not responsible for the reports from their respective areas. Perception of senior leadership as engaged and authoritative:

- reinforces commitment to the effort;
- focuses discussion on issues important to the overall goal;
- lends credibility to individuals exhibiting the behaviors and performance senior leadership desires;

- keeps senior leadership personally engaged and accountable; and
- keeps meetings brief and efficient.

Focus on Innovation

Not every participant in the 100-Day Quality Workout needs to stand up and present his or her results at each check-in. The executive champion and senior leaders should select individuals who have taken risks or used new strategies and methods. This highlight emphasizes the behaviors the organization desires and teaches critical lessons.

Updates delivered during the check-in should include the following information:

- Tests completed and change concepts applied
- Results from changes in work processes
- Lessons learned from tests
- Next steps for expansion or retesting
- Financial impact of changes

Summation/Kickoff

The summation/kickoff helps the organization maintain its momentum. It is a time to highlight individual or specific team efforts as well as examine the combined effort of all teams. It is also a time to have some fun, energize the group, and prepare them for the next round of activity.

The following three events compose the summation/kickoff:

- Abbreviated reporting of the most vital information
- Celebration of the total accomplishments of the 100-Day Quality Workout
- Kickoff of the next 100-Day Quality Workout

Abbreviated Status Reports

Reports for the summation/kickoff should follow the same pattern as those for the 30-, 60-, and 90-day check-ins, with two exceptions. First, the executive team leaders must be more selective in their reports to save time for the celebration event. Second, two hours should be reserved to educate participants on new tools and methods they will need in the upcoming 100-Day Quality Workout.

Summation Celebration

The summation celebration maintains momentum, keeps the quality system fresh, and increases staff morale. This event is a time for the group to summarize what it has accomplished and celebrate as a team. Executive leaders should include activities that recognize and reenergize team members. Injecting fun, humor, and an element of surprise prevents these meetings from becoming boring or tedious. Leaders have used the following types of awards and celebrations successfully.

- *Formal award ceremonies.* Gift certificates and awards are appropriate for those who have made significant contributions and accomplishments.
- *Quality waste Jeopardy.* Managers compete on their knowledge of the categories of waste and change concepts.
- *Parody of the Oscar ceremonies.* The executive champion wears a tuxedo and presents miniature statue awards, including awards for "Best Fiction," for a team whose numbers were exaggerated; "Best Drama," for a team that implemented a change that produced unintended consequences; and "Best Documentary," for a team that presented too many graphs and charts.
- *Traveling trophies.* Such awards create tradition, friendly rivalry, and competition.

Do what works for the specific culture of the hospital. Make the summation/kickoff an event that no manager wants to miss.

Do not limit your creativity. Structure recognition deliberately. Celebrate not only success but also failure when it results in learning and progress.

Kickoff for the Next 100-Day Quality Workout

Following the celebration phase, the executive champion should call a 15-minute break and then start the kickoff for the next 100-Day Quality Workout. Research shows that announcement of the focus of the next 100-Day Quality Workout at the summation/kickoff meeting is critical. Failure to do so generally results in a loss of momentum. Organizations can recover when they delay the launch of the next 100-Day Quality Workout by more than 30 days, but they lose precious time, and senior leaders must remotivate their teams. By immediately announcing the strategic focus and moving swiftly into the next 100-Day Quality Workout, senior leadership imbeds performance improvement in the culture as an ongoing quality system, not just a onetime project.

GAUGING YOUR CAPACITY FOR CHANGE

Every organization has a finite capacity for change. Cross this invisible barrier and performance improvement slows to a crawling pace or stops altogether. Because the 100-Day Quality Workout establishes a continuous process for performance improvement, senior leaders may not be aware of the total number and scope of performance improvement projects underway. Such lack of awareness may cause managers to engage in more initiatives than they can handle. Some of the most capable managers may be the ones who will take on new projects and not realize they have exceeded their capacity to improve. How can a senior leader determine when managers are approaching the tipping point?

Create a Centralized Improvement Projects Inventory

To get a comprehensive picture of their performance improvement initiatives, organizations should create a centralized improvement projects inventory. Advantages of such a tracking form include the ability to:

- link projects to larger core strategies;
- audit projects and halt those that are not useful;
- identify managers who are overtaxed or have reached their capacity for change; and
- gauge progress and identify slippage.

Resist the temptation to build an elaborate tool and collect extensive amounts of information. Such a system should include only basic information about a performance improvement project, including:

- a brief project description or name;
- links to organizational strategic initiatives;
- the person or team responsible for completing the project;
- the date the project was started;
- the target date for completion;
- the actual completion date;
- critical milestone dates;
- estimated return on investment or cost recovered; and
- validation by the finance department.

An accountability tracking system can be a simple tool residing in a Microsoft Excel spreadsheet linked by macros. Some organizations prefer to use a simple database in which managers can log their projects through standardized forms. A web-based platform is the best configuration because it provides updates on a real-time basis and is easily accessible from any computer in the organization. See Figure 3.2.

Figure 3.2 Example of Performance Improvement Tracking System

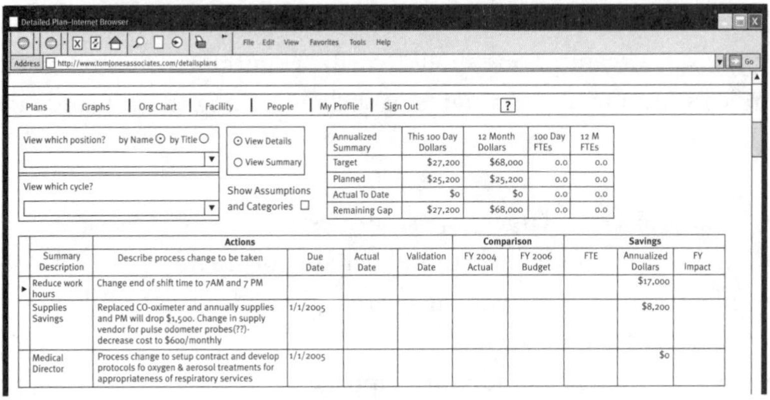

Annualized Summary	This 100 Day Dollars	12 Month Dollars	100 Day FTEs	12 M FTEs
Target	$27,200	$68,000	0.0	0.0
Planned	$25,200	$25,200	0.0	0.0
Actual To Date	$0	$0	0.0	0.0
Remaining Gap	$27,200	$68,000	0.0	0.0

Actions					Comparison		Savings		
Summary Description	Describe process change to be taken	Due Date	Actual Date	Validation Date	FY 2004 Actual	FY 2006 Budget	FTE	Annualized Dollars	FY Impact
Reduce work hours	Change end of shift time to 7AM and 7 PM							$17,000	
Supplies Savings	Replaced CO-oximeter and annually supplies and PM will drop $1,500. Change in supply vendor for pulse odometer probes(??)-decrease cost to $600/monthly	1/1/2005						$8,200	
Medical Director	Process change to setup contract and develop protocols fo oxygen & aerosol treatments for appropriateness of respiratory services	1/1/2005						$0	

We have observed many performance improvement and quality professionals who immediately want to expand the functionality of their tracking system and collect an increasing amount of data. Avoid this temptation and keep the system simple so the most computer-challenged clinical managers can enter their 100-day action plans in 20 minutes or less. Doing so will increase compliance and participation of staff.

Create a List of Projects That Are Not Useful

Central to the process is a quick periodic review by the senior leadership team to create a list of projects, teams, and committees that have outlived their usefulness (Caldwell 2008). If senior leaders sense that the organization is close to its capacity for change, they must remove or suspend something from the list before chartering a new initiative. At this time, senior leaders should take a critical look at all initiatives and see which are no longer relevant or necessary.

CONCLUSION

Top-performing organizations understand the need to make progress instantly visible. They know how to harness positive peer pressure and design tangible methods to foster accountability at every level. Using tools such as the 100-Day Quality Workout, senior leaders can maintain steady progress, detect slippage, and intervene before quality improvement veers off track.

REFERENCES

Caldwell, C. 2008. "Aggressively Improve Costs and Throughput Using Lean Six Sigma." Seminar presented by American College of Healthcare Executives, Keystone, CO, January 30–31.

Kotter, J. 1995. "Leading Change: Why Transformational Efforts Fail." *Harvard Business Review* 73 (2): 59–67.

Pieper, S. 2004. "'Good to Great' in Healthcare: How Some Organizations Are Elevating Their Performance." *Healthcare Executive* 19 (3): 20–26.

Stuenkel, K., and C. Caldwell. 2008. "The Senior Leader's Role in Improving Cost and Throughput." Presentation at Congress on Healthcare Leadership, Chicago, March 10–11.

Ulrich, D. 2002. *The GE Workout: How to Implement GE's Revolutionary Method for Busting Bureaucracy and Attacking Organizational Problems—Fast.* New York: McGraw-Hill.

CHAPTER 4

Linking Strategy
and Quality

*We are continually faced by great opportunities brilliantly dis-
guised as insoluble problems.*

—Lee Iaccoca

MANY SENIOR HEALTHCARE leaders have all but disengaged from the
quality process. These senior leaders believe quality plays a role in their
organization, but they do not see a connection between quality
improvement and the critical operating issues on which they focus the
majority of their attention, including bed capacity, declining reimbursement, physician relations, and operating margins. Organizations'
operating strategy and quality/performance improvement programs
never have aligned. As a result, many senior leaders have allowed their
quality departments and performance improvement teams to function
as monitors rather than drivers of meaningful change.

This lack of connection is unfortunate because quality directly
affects the bottom line of every healthcare institution. If an organization eliminates errors, waiting time, delays, and rework, shouldn't
some form of cost recovery result? If a hospital is staffed appropriately, shouldn't patient and staff satisfaction improve? If an organization uses advanced quality methods to improve patient flow,
shouldn't the hospital's capacity expand? Improving patient flow,

reducing wait times, and decreasing waste could generate increases in revenue, operating margin, and patient satisfaction and reduce the need for additional capital.

QUANTITY DOES NOT YIELD QUALITY

Many of the senior executive teams we encountered expressed that there is too much to do and not enough time to get it done. They have fewer resources to accomplish more, in less time. Consumed by the urgent matters of the day, senior executives ignore strategic imperatives. Some track dozens of projects, task forces, and committees, whereas others only speculate on the full scope and breadth of their chartered work teams.

When we questioned these senior leaders about tangible results, the conversation usually slowed and sometimes halted completely. They chartered many of their projects without a strategic framework. They initiated these projects because of an urgent need rather than because of a strategically important imperative. At best, these organizations' efforts are a collection of unrelated projects with no cohesive strategic direction. These performance improvement initiatives even may be working at cross-purposes. They work to optimize the performance of a single department rather than overall hospital performance.

Having a long list of projects does not equate to being highly productive and progressive. Senior executives often delegate and deploy every available ounce of the organization's capacity to transform processes, but this approach fails to account for an organization's limited capacity for change. Once an organization's threshold for change is crossed, every new initiative is another brick on the wagon that bogs down the managers and pushes them another step beyond their capacity to engage in meaningful work.

Organizations weighted down by a random approach to performance improvement do not recognize the liberating effects of strategic focus. Many senior leaders believe they have established strategic performance improvement goals. They often proclaim a broad performance improvement goal of "improving patient satisfaction from 75 percent to 90 percent" or "lowering the cost of patient care per adjusted patient day or discharge by 5 percent." These goal statements are ineffective because they do not explain how the organization will achieve the goal and what role senior leaders will assume in the process. Such goals are more effective when restated in terms of process changes that communicate the path to success and reduce it to tangible behaviors. For example, the first goal could be restated as, "Our hospital will improve patient satisfaction by designing work processes that ensure every emergency room patient is seen by a physician in 30 minutes or less." The second goal could be restated as, "We will reduce our operating expenses by 10 percent by improving our staffing processes such that we achieve our definition of quality staffing 95 percent of the time." These restated goals connect the broader goals of patient satisfaction and lower operating costs with specific processes. In other words, they link strategy with quality improvement and provide clear guidance on the process elements that require improvement.

DEFINING YOUR CORE PROCESSES

Quantum improver organizations understand the importance of linking operating strategies to their quality efforts. They have a clear sense of core work processes integral to the organization's operational success and understand that quality improvement in these major core processes will result in improved clinical outcomes, financial performance, and patient satisfaction.

Eliyahu Goldratt and the Theory of Constraints
Eliyahu Goldratt (1984), who developed the Theory of Constraints and laid the foundations for Lean methodology, understood the importance of focus and vision when he wrote *The Goal: A Process of Ongoing Improvement*. This best-selling book is set in the context of an industrial

---

(Continued on following page)

(Continued from previous page)

plant that has gone through extensive investments in automation. The central character is faced with a perplexing question. Although the plant is exceeding all productivity measures by the company's accounting standards and each production step is achieving the company's highest measures of productivity, it is losing money. Why? The answer and solution are revealed as the general manager asks a simple but important question: "What is our goal: to optimize the efficiency of each department or to ship billable inventory off the loading dock?" This question brought focus and clarity to the organization, which needed to redesign its work processes. It realized that its ultimate goal was to ship completed inventory off the dock, not to optimize the performance of each department.

Senior leaders must take an in-depth look at this fundamental question: What is our goal, and what are the core processes that will determine our success? Hospital employees often are engaged in improving the performance of their departments, yet they lack a fundamental understanding of how their efforts will improve the hospital's overall performance.

How does an organization determine what its core processes are, and where should it focus its attention? An organization's work processes can be divided into two categories: (1) strategic work processes, or as we like to call them, "Big Quality" or "Big Q" core processes, and (2) sub-processes, or "little q" processes. Big Q core processes are integral to an organization's overall performance and represent areas on which an organization should focus its quality efforts. Little q processes, although important, often are sub-processes of Big Q core processes.

In their book *Lean-Six Sigma for Healthcare*, Caldwell, Brexler, and Gillem (2005) propose a framework that hospital executives can use to determine and create metrics for their Big Q core processes. The following questions test whether a core process is truly strategic.

- Is the process significant enough to warrant a performance improvement or quality improvement project at all times, over many years, because it is based on the organization's strategic and operational needs?

- Does this process "define" the healthcare organization, and does it address the essence of why the organization exists and what it does?
- Is this process measured by trending toward a goal over time?
- Would performance improvement in this area be owned by a senior leader or delegated to a junior leader or manager?
- Is this process significant enough that failure to achieve the desired improvement or goal would have serious consequences for the organization?

Although Big Q core processes vary among organizations, the following list represents some common core processes identified by quantum improver organizations and other organizations we studied. The list has been reviewed by thousands of senior healthcare leaders with a high degree of consensus. Not everyone has to agree with each item on this list, but every leadership team should take the time to develop its own prioritized list. Using this list as a starting point may generate ideas and stimulate conversation.

- *Effective staffing.* The largest and most expensive work process for any healthcare provider is its staffing process. Most executives have not considered staffing as a work process, yet every department has a work process it uses to have the right person in the right place at the right time. In most healthcare organizations, the staffing work process influences approximately 50 percent of the organization's total fiscal budget. In addition, the staffing process affects just about every other aspect of hospital performance, such as quality of care, patient satisfaction, wait times, and patient throughput.
- *Patient flow through the emergency department.* The emergency department is the front door to most hospitals and a major source of admissions. It is also the beginning of the patient's experience with the hospital. A patient's dissatisfaction with

his or her experience in the emergency department is likely to taint the patient's evaluation of his or her entire experience. This negative halo effect presents a service recovery challenge for every other department in the hospital.

- *Patient flow through the surgical department.* Surgery represents one of the main service lines of most hospitals and is a significant source of operating margin. In addition, surgery tends to be one of the most expensive and resource-intensive work processes.

- *Patient discharge cycle.* In many healthcare markets, bed capacity is at a premium. Executives are facing the choice of improving their existing capacity or seeking capital expansion to meet the needs of their communities. The patient discharge cycle and admission of the next patient directly influence bed capacity. Senior leaders must think of this process as a cycle because value is generated only when the next patient is admitted.

- *Use of clinical core measures.* Over the past 20 years, managed healthcare organizations, the Centers for Medicare & Medicaid Services (CMS), and others have spent billions of dollars on research and data analysis to determine appropriate levels of care and the most efficacious treatments. Although there can be reasonable disagreement with some of their decisions, particularly when reimbursement is at stake, in aggregate these measures provide an excellent guideline by which to examine the quality of clinical practices.

- *Revenue cycle accuracy.* Organizations can use the accuracy of their revenue cycle as a primary measure of how well they are reimbursed for the care they provide. They can gain or lose significant money depending on the efficiency and accuracy of their revenue cycle.

MAKING THE BIG Q LIST MANAGEABLE

One critical point to remember is that any list of Big Q core processes should be manageable, and organizations should resist the temptation to expand the list too much. Consider how many items you can remember from a long list. When listening to a speech, at what number of points do you lose track of the speaker's message? Most people can remember no more than seven points. Assume that you succumb to the temptation of increasing your list of core processes to ten, under which you add another ten sub-processes. How will your staff know which are the most important?

DETERMINING BIG Q CORE METRICS

Once an organization has determined its core processes, it must associate a metric with each core process to help quantify improvement. Big Q core processes are exponentially more effective when senior executives explicitly define what they mean by "quality" and incorporate measurable elements of the work processes critical to success. To be useful as a Big Q core metric, values must be specific and stated in terms of upper and lower standards of performance.

The following sections discuss possible metrics for the Big Q core processes we identified. These work processes and associated metrics may not be appropriate for every organization, but they do represent areas on which many quantum improver organizations have focused their quality improvement efforts.

Effective Staffing

An organization is "in quality" with regard to staffing when it is achieving its own standards of quality staffing 95 percent of the time. Few healthcare providers have taken the step to define what they mean by "quality staffing." Some hospitals and professional associations have set upper specification limits (USLs), such as patient-to-nurse ratios, but few have applied the same diligence in establishing corresponding lower specification limits (LSLs). An organization is just as "out of quality" when it has too few patients per nurse as when it has too many. Staffing that exceeds patient demand is a form of quality waste. In this situation, the organization could have used these valuable resources elsewhere.

Setting an upper and lower specification limit is important when determining quality staffing. For example, a nursing unit can define itself as achieving in-quality staffing levels when the unit has no more than six patients per nurse but no fewer than three patients per nurse. The unit is in quality when it is within the bounds of these upper and lower specification limits.

Figure 4.1 illustrates the concept of in-quality staffing. In this example, the emergency department nurse manager defined "in quality" as no more than six patients (the USL) but no fewer than three patients (the LSL) assigned to one nurse. The manager set a strategic goal of meeting her own definition of quality staffing 95 percent of the time. In other words, 95 percent of the time, the nursing staff has three or more patients, but no more than six patients, assigned to one nurse.

The x-axis represents the hours of the day, beginning at 7 a.m. The framework of this view of quality is centered on the y-axes. The left axis indicates volume per hour, and the right axis notates the volume per

Figure 4.1 An Emergency Department Manager's In-Quality Staffing Analysis

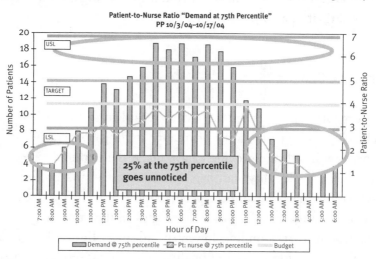

What Top-Performing Healthcare Organizations Know

staff person per hour. The USL and LSL frame the manager's definition of quality. A line that reflects the department at budget also may be added to the graph. In Figure 4.1, the budget rests approximately at four patients per nurse. The nursing manager would have an affordance of two patients. An *affordance* is the level of variation a department can manage, beyond which it would encounter problems with quality. In other words, the department in Figure 4.1 is budgeted for four patients per nurse, but for short periods it can accommodate variation ranging from two to six patients per nurse.

Figure 4.2 illustrates a radiology department manager's in-quality staffing analysis. In this manager's opinion, a radiology technologist is "in quality" when he or she is scheduled to perform between six and eight exams per hour.

Benefits to the in-quality staffing approach are numerous. This staffing strategy is based on a quality approach rather than external productivity standards or benchmarks, which invite arguments from managers. Benchmarks and productivity standards tell the manager nothing about what needs to change in the work or care processes.

Figure 4.2 Example of Radiology Department Manager's In-Quality Staffing Analysis

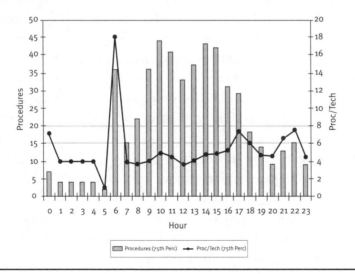

In contrast, the in-quality staffing approach allows managers to define quality, use their own data, develop their own master staffing plans, and pinpoint which element of the staffing process needs to be changed. Consequently, this approach tends to reduce resistance to change and thus increases the hospital's speed to action.

Consider an Hour-by-Hour Staffing Approach

Big Q Metric: Achieve In-Quality Staffing More than 95 Percent of the Time

Senior leaders, particularly the chief nurse executive, find it difficult to engage nursing managers in staffing examinations. Nursing managers feel that they already have worked hard to recruit and retain nursing staff and that further optimization is unnecessary. When confronted with the prospect of altering their current staffing plans, managers inevitably raise concerns about negatively affecting quality.

Most healthcare organizations' staffing strategies are based on relatively static plans or on 12-hour shifts. Unfortunately, quality does not come in even 12-hour blocks. Managers often build their staffing plans on the basis of perceptions and customs rather than on an objective analysis of patient demand or units of service. A manager's perception of demand is unreliable as a planning tool because it often exaggerates busy times and peak workloads. Likewise, slower times and decreased demand go unnoticed. Managers often react with surprise the first time they see a statistically valid analysis of how their actual staffing compares to demand.

Instead of viewing staffing from a 12- or 24-hour perspective, organizations should consider conducting a statistically valid assessment of department demand on an hour-by-hour basis. When hour-by-hour workload is analyzed side by side with hour-by-hour staffing, managers, particularly nurse managers, become excited because this method of staffing analysis uncovers quality problems endemic to their day-to-day frustrations. As managers balance the hour-by-hour staffing as it relates to hour-by-hour volume, they find that they not only have more staff than they realized but that they need less staff.

Emergency Department/Bed Management

Big Q Metric: Emergency Department Length of Stay of Less than Three Hours to Home Discharge or Four Hours or Less to Hospital Admission

Length of stay (LOS) and time to admission in the emergency department are two indicators of quality of patient care in the emergency department. Remember that variation, not average LOS, creates patient dissatisfaction. Patients reach a point after which their LOS becomes unacceptable. As a recommendation, consider metrics that indicate that no patient discharged to home should have an LOS longer than three hours, and if admitted, the LOS should not exceed four hours. Real gains occur only when we view this metric within the continuum of departments that work with the emergency department, including bed management and the other ancillary departments involved in patient flow. Organizations must consider what occurs in the laboratory department, radiology department, patient transport function, bed request process, and other critical inputs. These sub-process drivers influence total LOS and "left without treatment" rates.

Several sub-processes within the organization may affect LOS and should be considered in quality efforts. We compiled the following list of critical sub-processes from the analysis of multiple emergency departments (Caldwell 2008).

Sub-Process	Critical Metric
Walk-in to emergency department bed	<30 minutes
Emergency department bed to emergency department physician assessment	<15 minutes
Time to last diagnostic order	<45 minutes

Lab/X-ray order to results	<15 minutes
Diagnostic result to emergency department physician review	<15 minutes
Bed notified to transport	<30 minutes
Discharge order to discharge	<20 minutes
In-quality staffing	>95 percent
Emergency department physician variation	<25 percent

Surgery Cut-to-Close Time

Big Q Metric: Total Surgical Hours Are More than 40 Percent of Staffed Hours

Comparison of surgery cut-to-close time to staffing time provides a global measure of the percentage of time the surgical department is doing what it is paid to do. The surgery cut-to-close measurement is an accurate reflection of the percentage of labor committed to delivering surgical services. By definition, it can never be greater than 50 percent because the minimum staffing for the operating room consists of a surgical nurse and a circulator. At the surgical department's most efficient state, it achieves one minute of surgical time for every two minutes of labor, thus limiting the measure at all times to no more than 50 percent. From the perspective of the payer and the patient, the actual surgery is the only value-added step in the work process. Pre- and post-operation activities are important and necessary but considered business value added or non-value added (waste). A surgical staff's natural reaction is to want to count only what actually occurs from the start of the surgery until close. However, experience indicates that most waste and opportunity arise in the work processes that occur before and after the operating room procedure. As a senior executive, you should examine and consider as much of the surgical-related labor component as possible to identify the maximum amount of waste and opportunity. As a Big Q metric, surgery cut-to-close time highlights this pre- and post-waste.

Surgery cut-to-close hours can be calculated by dividing operating room hours by operating room staffed hours. The higher the percentage of operating room staff time spent performing surgery rather than other tasks, the more efficient the department is.

The ideal capacity metric would be surgery cut-to-close hours divided by the number of hours the operating rooms are available for scheduling. However, we have found that available hours data, as downloaded from surgery legacy systems, are often inaccurate. Worked hours data, easily recoverable from the payroll system, are more reliable.

As with the emergency department, there are several sub-processes in the surgery department that affect surgery cut-to-close time and staff hours. The following list of sub-process metrics correlates directly with accurate surgical start time and efficient work processes in the operating room.

Sub-Process	Critical Metric
Incision time no later than	<7:40 a.m. start time
Room turnaround time	<15 minutes
Variance or delay to next case	+/−15 minutes
Surgeon preference card accuracy	>95 percent
Surgeon in-room to scheduled time	+/−15 minutes

Discharge Cycle

Big Q Metric: Patient Discharged by 2 p.m. and Bed Turnaround to Next Patient Within 60 Minutes More than 80 Percent of the Time
Another quality metric is the percentage of time the hospital discharges a patient and moves the next patient into the bed on a timely basis. The suggested Big Q metric is a greater than 80 percent occurrence of a 2 p.m. discharge and bed turnaround to the next patient within 60 minutes. Most hospitals are working on initiatives to improve their discharge processes, but many fail to view this process as a cycle. Patient discharge time alone insufficiently measures quality and performance if organizations leave

needed beds unfilled because of gaps in their discharge processes. In our research, nursing staff frequently expressed frustration that the physicians did not write all discharge orders by 7:30 a.m. These nurses failed to realize that chaos would have resulted if they had done so because the hospital did not have the resources to discharge all the patients at one time. An appointment or slotting system is a logical alternative. Substantial gains are achievable only when staff realizes that discharge appointments are necessary to smooth out workflow and prevent bottlenecks in the patient discharge process. When a discharge appointment is missed, it is gone forever.

The following list of sub-process metrics indicates a well-engineered discharge cycle.

Sub-Process	Critical Metric
Zero missed discharge appointments	Discharge within 30 minutes of appointment
Physician review of last lab results	<4 hours before discharge
Transportation confirmation	Before 4 p.m. previous day

Revenue Cycle Accuracy

Big Q Metric: Greater than 75 Percent Clean Claims Submitted

Most healthcare organizations look at accounts receivable as a primary measure of how well their organization receives reimbursement for the care it provides. To measure the efficiency of this process, organizations can look at the percentage of clean claims. The Big Q metric is 75 percent clean claims within five days post-discharge. The following sub-processes drive accuracy.

Sub-Process	Critical Metric
Coding accuracy	>95 percent
Documentation available for billing	>95 percent

| Clean claims post-discharge | <5 days |
| Claims paid in x days post-discharge | >80 percent |

Clinical Core Measures

Big Q Metric: Clinical Core Measure: 0 Percent Denial of Reimbursement for Patient Care

None of the other Big Q core processes evokes more discussion and debate among senior leaders than selection of a Big Q metric for clinical core measure. One logical metric is the percentage of patient care denied for reimbursement. The logic behind selection of this measure is as follows: Measure the percentage of time a hospital matches a universally accepted definition or its own definition of quality healthcare. The key is to establish a definition of what constitutes quality care and what care the hospital will provide. Ideally, this care should match the care for which the hospital will be reimbursed. For a place to start in determining appropriate care and defining quality, we suggest examining the guidelines established by CMS and other payer sources. CMS, health maintenance organizations, and other payers have invested considerable resources and research to identify appropriate levels of patient care. One strategy for measuring clinical effectiveness in Lean-Six Sigma terms is to track the percentage of time the organization is meeting its definition of quality care based on accepted practices. This approach does not obligate the hospital to use external standards of care. The hospital can use them, however, as a starting point for creating its own standards. If there are disagreements about the external standards, the hospital can modify the definitions and create an affordance, or planned variation. This approach uses a quality-based method of tracking the care provided. This large metric assesses need for the care provided, documentation for payment, and the probability that the hospital will receive reimbursement for the care it provided.

LINKING BIG Q PROCESSES TO PERFORMANCE IMPROVEMENT

Once an organization has gained consensus on its top Big Q core processes and associated metrics, senior leaders should determine whether performance improvement projects underway in the organization are improving the Big Q core metrics.

The following exercise provides an assessment of the strategic importance of the organization's current portfolio of performance improvement initiatives. It also reveals which of the organization's current projects are critical to its operational performance.

Senior leaders also should consider Big Q core processes when choosing a focus for a 100-Day Quality Workout. Because of the size and scope of a Big Q core process, a typical 100-Day Quality Workout should focus on one or maybe two sub-processes of a Big Q core process. We recommend the following questions as selection guidelines.

1. Which one or two Big Q core processes do we need to improve in the next 100 days?
2. Do we have actionable information, data, or analysis to support our answer to question 1? Sources may include inherent departmental information ("tribal knowledge"), best practice databases, consulting reports, Healthcare Advisory Board reports, and professional association reports.
3. Do we believe we have identified at least some of our critical sub-processes because of the staff's current knowledge? What is the probability that this actionable information will yield an improvement?
4. Do the benefits of taking action today outweigh the benefits of inaction?

There are times when a team needs new insights to rejuvenate its efforts and make progress. Chapter 6 discusses the statistical tools and analytical processes of quality improvement tools, such as Lean and Six Sigma, that offer such valuable insights.

CONCLUSION

By linking performance improvement to an organization's Big Q core processes, senior leaders can ensure that they direct work to the most critical areas of an organization. Changes that lead to operational and quality improvements will reinforce the concept that performance improvement is continuous.

REFERENCES

Caldwell, C. 2008. "Aggressively Improve Costs and Throughput Using Lean Six Sigma." Seminar presented by American College of Healthcare Executives, Keystone, CO, January 30–31.

Caldwell, C., J. Brexler, and T. Gillem. 2005. *Lean-Six Sigma for Healthcare: A Senior Leader Guide to Improving Cost and Throughput*. Milwaukee, WI: Quality Press.

Goldratt, E. 1984. *The Goal: A Process of Ongoing Improvement*. Great Barrington, MA: North River Press.

CHAPTER 5

Creating an Environment
for Change

The rate of change is not going to slow down anytime soon. If anything, competition in most industries will probably speed up even more in the next few decades.

—John P. Kotter

AN ENVIRONMENT OF change does not just materialize. An organization creates such an environment through a deliberate series of actions to pave the way for future success. Creating an environment of change is the equivalent of tilling the soil in preparation for planting. The soil, or environment, must contain the right ingredients if seeds are to germinate and develop into a harvestable crop. In addition to a strong accountability system, several ingredients are essential to creating a healthy environment for change:

- Clarity of vision and focus
- Effective communication about vision and focus
- Cultural characteristics that promote and reward change

CLARITY OF VISION AND FOCUS

Hospital employees often work to improve the performance of their departments but lack a fundamental understanding of how their efforts will affect the overall performance of the hospital. Without a clear vision from senior leadership, individual employees and teams are left to answer a variety of questions about what needs to change and how they will accomplish those changes. Senior leaders must take deliberate actions to frame the discussion and answer some of the following key questions.

- Why must changes be made now?
- How will these changes contribute to the organization's larger performance goals, and what is the ultimate goal?
- What are the metrics by which we will define success?
- What will we improve?
- How will we improve it?
- How will making the proposed changes affect stakeholders?

Lack of clarity on these issues may result in confusion concerning priorities and dissipate efforts as people affected by the change pursue different solutions. For example, assume you are a director of radiology. Is your goal to run the most efficient and effective imaging department or to play a role in the hospital's larger goals of decreasing emergency department wait times and improving bed capacity? How you view your goal has a profound effect on which projects you will select and metrics you will track to measure success. If your goal is to run the most efficient radiology department, you will choose batch processing and design workflows that may sub-optimize total patient flow. Unintentionally, batching of results will create extended wait times and a bottleneck of work downstream.

Establishing a Clear Vision Statement

Employees in quantum improver organizations have a strong sense of why the organization exists and feel a sense of urgency in supporting the organization's destiny. An organization's vision statement helps convey this sense of purpose and establish this sense of urgency. Such a statement must comprise more than basic platitudes such as "provide world-class care" and explicitly state the organization's goals and the "who, what, where, why, and how" of achieving them.

What Composes an Effective Vision Statement?

Most hospitals can point to an attractive slogan-style vision statement hanging in their lobby. Most statements express nebulous goals such as to "provide the best care" or "achieve service excellence." These global vision statements may produce warm feelings, but they provide the department manager with limited instructive value about how to achieve performance goals. Such statements do not relate to the manager's daily work or to the organization's larger strategic goals. Goals are exponentially more effective when senior executives explicitly define what they mean by quality and incorporate measurable elements of work processes critical to success.

An effective vision statement conveys deep, gut-level direction on how a department is to support the hospital's core processes. The statement is as brief as possible without omitting details required to communicate the vision effectively.

We developed the following list of key questions to help senior leaders focus their vision statements to a concise document that helps managers understand their role and objectives in the change process. Answers to the following questions translate a strong vision statement into actionable steps (Caldwell 2008).

- Which Big Q core processes are vital to the organization's success?
- Which Big Q core processes are the focus of the organization, and in what order will they be improved during the next three years?
- Why must the organization make changes to these Big Q core processes now?
- How will we measure success with our Big Q core processes?
- How do we define quality service and care? What sub-processes will affect success?
- How do we define quality in terms of sub-process metrics?
- Who will benefit from our Big Q core process initiatives? Patients? Community? Physicians? Clinical staff? Employees?
- How will major stakeholders benefit?
  - Improved cost recovery?
  - Expanded capacity to deliver care?
  - Reduced wait times for patients?
  - Increased satisfaction of employees and medical staff?
  - Preserved capital for other critical needs?
- What possible objections, concerns, and points of confusion do we anticipate in moving forward with our work?

By establishing clear goals to transform work processes, senior leaders can begin to break down silo thinking. Such goals force me, as a department manager, to examine how my work supports the hospital's larger core processes. Establishing clear goals is the first step toward ensuring that incentives are aligned and preventing Kotter's (1995) error 2: not creating a powerful enough guiding coalition.

Figure 5.1 is an executive guide for developing a strong vision statement.

Following is a fictitious example of how senior leaders can cascade the traditional mission statement into specific areas of focus for each department. Note how these statements focus managers' attention on the role their department plays in the organization's

Figure 5.1 Executive Leader's Vision Assessment

	Strategic Component	Question
1	Strategic alignment	Is our performance improvement vision aligned with our strategic operational goals?
		Is our vision consistent with other communications, priorities, mandates, and goals?
		Is our vision statement consistent with the organization's values?
		Is our vision internally consistent, with few contradictions or conflicts?
2	Focus	Does the vision provide managers with a clear focus on the work processes and sub-processes vital to the organization's success?
3	Sense of urgency	Does our vision statement clearly explain why this change is necessary?
4	Interest of stakeholders	Does the statement clearly identify the benefits that will accrue to each stakeholder if the initiative is successful?
		Have we crafted appropriate messages that speak to each stakeholder?
5	Clarity	Is the statement clear and easy to understand?
6	Process changes	Does the vision provide a clear understanding of which core processes will be the focus of the organization's efforts?
7	Skills and knowledge	Does the vision articulate the specific skills, training, or knowledge that process owners must have to succeed in the transformational effort?

strategy and the direction they provide on how to design the department's work processes.

Hospital level: For 120 years, Memorial Hospital's mission has been to advance the health and well-being of people in the community in partnership with those it serves. The hospital works to achieve outstanding performance through patient care, education, and outreach that offer high-quality, advanced technology and exceptional service to support patients and their families. As part of its mission, Memorial Hospital is committed to providing the highest-quality emergency department care in the city by achieving the following standard of performance:

Big Q metric for emergency department services: All emergency department patients will be discharged in less than three hours or admitted in no more than four hours.

Department level: Sub-process drivers: The emergency department will design its work processes to achieve the following levels of service:

- Every patient will be greeted within five minutes of arrival at the emergency department.
- No patient will wait more than 30 minutes to see a physician and receive an emergency department bed.
- The lab will make available, and physicians will strive to review and write, orders within 45 minutes after the last diagnostic test was ordered.
- Lab and X-ray results will be available within 60 minutes of their order.
- No more than 15 minutes will elapse from the time a bed is available until the patient is transported.
- The emergency department will be at in-quality staffing levels of greater than 95 percent every day.

A clear statement defining quality and levels of service focuses the organization on vital parts of its work processes. Taking the time to answer the questions in Figure 5.1 is an excellent way to avoid Kotter's (1995) error 3: lacking a vision.

COMMUNICATING YOUR VISION AND FOCUS WITH CLARITY

Senior leaders must communicate the vision through every appropriate channel. Communicating the vision should not be taken for granted nor considered a onetime event. They should communicate the vision constantly and consistently and revisit it to make sure that it fits the evolving environment.

Many senior leaders mistakenly think that communicating the vision once is enough. The moment they begin to tire of repeating the message, however, may be the moment it is beginning to sink in. To avoid Kotter's (1995) error 4—undercommunicating by a factor of ten—senior leaders must assume a campaign mentality and realize that winning the hearts and minds of the staff is a long-term battle.

CULTURAL CHARACTERISTICS THAT PROMOTE CHANGE

In addition to clear visions and goals, critical factors must be present within an organization's culture for change initiatives to be successful. Employees across the organization must be comfortable with change, have a bias toward action, and feel confident about trying new initiatives instead of fearing failure.

Assessing Organizational Comfort with Change

Change is inevitable. Organizations that do not embrace change are destined to fail. How does your organization rate? How comfortable are your employees with change? Do they feel empowered to make changes? If you came to work as a manager in your organization tomorrow, would a portion of your job be dedicated to improving work processes? Would taking calculated risks and proactively driving needed change enhance your self-esteem, or would you learn that the best path to career longevity is to keep a low profile and maintain the status quo? The following questions are designed to prompt an honest introspective discussion of whether your hospital's culture fosters an expectation of change.

- Cultural expectation of change
  - Have we explicitly stated the expectation that a percentage of a manager's job is dedicated to performance improvement?
  - Has performance improvement been integrated into compensation?
  - Is successfully managing transformational efforts a prerequisite for promotion to a larger role?
- Systematic approach to recognize initiative
  - Do we have a formal process for recognizing managers who take calculated risks?
  - Do we informally and personally recognize those who exhibit the traits we desire?
  - Do we have a formal process to identify individuals who have led successful change?
- Eliminating cultural barriers to change
  - Are there punitive barriers, either implicit or explicit, that protect the status quo?

By answering these questions honestly, the senior team can prevent Kotter's (1995) error 5: not removing the obstacles to the new vision.

Assessing an Organization's Tolerance for Failure

Fear can immobilize any project or change initiative that has an element of risk or ambiguity. Because all transformational work produces false starts, unintended results, and even failure, those who venture outside their comfort zones to test changes in work processes will experience setbacks and failures. In the healthcare environment, failure generally is not tolerated or rewarded. Creative thinking and risk taking often is squelched. To achieve success, organizations must allow and even reward employees for taking risks to improve performance. The following questions can help you evaluate your organization's acceptance of risk.

- Clear boundaries governing change have been established.
  - Have senior executives explicitly set out rules or boundaries governing how managers can test changes?
  - Do managers operating within the guidelines have immunity and freedom from negative repercussions when testing changes in work processes?
- Senior leaders celebrate failure.
  - Do senior executives recognize and formally reward those who take calculated risks?
  - Do senior executives showcase momentary failures critical to the organization's ultimate achievement of performance gains?
- Managers manifest experimental thinking.
  - Are managers encouraged to test changes in work processes on a small scale before implementing changes on a permanent basis?
  - Do managers incrementally build belief in the new work processes, or do they believe they need unanimous agreement before implementing a change?
- Senior leaders promote an environment where small tests of change are welcomed.
  - When managers offer potential solutions, do senior leaders actively encourage them to test their ideas?
  - Do senior leaders coach actively, and are they skilled in the design of experiments?

Assessing an Organization's Bias Toward Action

A bias toward action is one of the most critical characteristics of organizations that achieve transformational results. Most healthcare organizations tend to be biased against speed and are focused on planning, data analysis, and careful implementation only after all possible issues are addressed. How does your organization rate? Does your organization lean toward dependence on scheduled meetings, formal approval processes, and excessive team participation, or are your managers biased toward spontaneous decisions, impromptu meetings, and SWOT (strengths, weaknesses, opportunities, and threats) team structures? Do department managers need formal approval before making changes, or are they empowered to act on their own as long as they keep management informed? The following questions can help you assess your organization's bias toward action.

- "Do now" mind-set
  - Do managers immediately take action when there are changes that can be made today?
  - Are impromptu meetings encouraged to avoid unnecessary delays in progress?
- Dealing with ambiguity
  - Are teams immobilized by perpetual analysis?
  - Is there a tendency for the discussion in meetings to focus on unknown information instead of actionable, available information?
- Expectation of action
  - Is there an expectation that every team meeting will result in initiation of some formal action or improvement?
  - Do teams have defined periods in which analysis and planning end, and action and implementation begin?
- Parallel processing
  - Do managers have the skills and training to break complex problems into solvable tasks, or are they likely to be overwhelmed by the scope of needed changes?

- Are teams working on projects in a linear manner, solving each problem sequentially, or are they working on parallel tracks?
- Does all work stop when the team identifies a roadblock, or does the team focus on the parts of the project that can move forward?

Achieving Speed to Action

The ability to achieve speed to action is one of the most critical elements in creating an environment for change. It involves quickly setting goals, overcoming the fear of change, and establishing processes that promote change. The following techniques and methods are commonly used to achieve speed to action.

- Avoid benchmarking unless you need it to identify opportunities or convince a group of the need to change. When you do need it, have a large and aggressive peer group assess the amount of opportunity.
- Set performance improvement goals quickly. Establish goals in 30 days or less to maintain momentum. If using benchmark data to set a goal, establish the goal at 50 percent or less of the performance gap between your organization and the benchmark. Setting the goal at 100 percent of the gap generally results in staff resistance and arguments about the accuracy of the data.
- Separate goal setting from the identification of solutions. If managers tie the two steps together, they may focus more on solutions that will not work rather than on how to achieve a desired goal effectively.

Promote Rapid Cycle Testing
Rapid cycle testing (RCT) is one of the most effective tools executive leaders have for accelerating change (Langley et al. 1996).

Thomas Noland, an international leader in applying statistics to healthcare, developed this concept. The idea behind RCT is that organizations can design an experiment that incrementally tests a proposed change over one or two shifts until there is sufficient evidence that the change has improved the process. Once improvement is realized, the change can be rolled out across a larger portion of the organization.

As managers make changes, they often have fears about patient satisfaction, physician complaints, or strain on employees. RCTs create a safe and controlled environment in which managers quickly can see whether their fears are real or imagined. For example, if staff and managers are saying, "We will never get all the doctors to agree to this change," the RCT method would encourage them to say, "Can we gain the support of one or two of the physicians to try the change during the next shift?"

RCT saves valuable time by quickly ruling out an experimental solution showing limited promise. RCT also detects unintended consequences and allows the organization to make adjustments. It allows organizations to refine each sub-process of a larger problem rather than implement multiple changes simultaneously and hope everything works flawlessly.

Consequently, RCT provides executive leaders with small wins that keep their performance improvement teams motivated and lead to greater progress. The concept of RCT addresses Kotter's (1995) error 6: not planning for and creating short-term wins.

A failed rapid cycle test is often more informative than a successful rapid cycle test because it is indicative of a hidden or unknown variable. Instead of a failure, it should be viewed as a rich learning opportunity to discover an important variable in the work process that the work team had not considered previously. This discovery moves the team one step closer to a workable solution. By its very nature, RCT promotes the belief that failure is not the final judgment but rather a step to learning what will work. The team does not stop trying but uses failure to learn and try another approach. Ultimately, RCT builds support for change.

CONCLUSION

Building an environment of change does not happen overnight. It requires dedication and continued vigilance. The good news is that using an established accountability system, linking strategy to quality, clearly establishing and communicating organizational visions and goals, and moving the organization to action can help transform the culture into one in which change efforts thrive and performance improvement is routine.

REFERENCES

Caldwell, C. 2008. "Aggressively Improve Costs and Throughput Using Lean Six Sigma." Seminar presented by American College of Healthcare Executives, Keystone, CO, January 30–31.

Kotter, J. 1995. "Leading Change: Why Transformational Efforts Fail." *Harvard Business Review* 73 (2): 59–67.

Langley, G. J., K. M. Nolan, T. W. Nolan, C. L. Norman, and L. P. Provost. 1996. *The Improvement Guide*. San Francisco: Jossey-Bass.

CHAPTER 6

Using Advanced Quality Methods

Quality is not an act, it is a habit.

—Aristotle (384 B.C.–322 B.C.)

TRAINING STAFF IN advanced quality methods without providing a framework and accountability system in which to apply these methods will produce suboptimal results. Senior executives must remember that quality methods are secondary to a strong accountability system and environment of change, but in the right context, they can accelerate progress of performance improvement activities. Every quality system eventually will optimize its results, but periodic injections of advanced quality methods will keep your program vibrant and maintain momentum.

INTRODUCING NEW METHODS AND TOOLS

Many executive leadership teams believe that their quality system and managers' skills are already optimal. Managers have exhausted their current set of skills for improving work processes. Asking them to reduce their full-time equivalent staff by another 5 percent or more is not a sustainable approach. Achieving additional gains in performance will require the introduction of new methods, tools, and skills.

Which methods and tools are appropriate? Across the healthcare industry, senior leaders are debating which set of advanced quality methods best tackles today's challenges. Some hospitals have implemented Lean methodology and are realizing significant gains in performance. Others have embraced Six Sigma and can offer evidence of significant reductions in emergency department wait times or increased surgical capacity. Which is the best method? The appropriate and truthful answer to this question depends on the circumstances. No quality acceleration method is superior to another. A claim of method superiority is as logical as saying a hammer or a screwdriver is the best tool for all projects. Eventually, all the tools will be needed. Each of these methods must be considered in the context of the organization's immediate improvement needs, its culture, and its staff's skill level.

AN OVERVIEW OF THE OPTIONS

Plan-Do-Check-Act

Plan-Do-Check-Act (PDCA) (or Plan-Do-Study-Act [PDSA]) evolved out of concepts initially framed by Shewhart in 1939 and was originally intended to create "a dynamic scientific process of acquiring knowledge" about quality issues and other problems (Bradbury 2008). Japanese quality circles incorporated PDCA in the 1950s and 1960s. A description of its components follows.

- Plan
  - Determine goals
  - Determine methods of reaching goals
- Do
  - Engage in education and training
  - Initiate implementation of work

- Check
  - Check the effects of implementation
- Act
  - Take appropriate actions

Later, Deming expanded on Shewhart's work by proposing that to "check" understates the value of learning that can occur. The term *check* implies confirmation that the variable is within specifications only. Deming advocated a more robust step that others began to call "study." Deming realized that it was important not only to assess quality but also to seek a deeper understanding about what was occurring in the process. The steps involved in Deming's approach follow.

- Plan
  - Plan a change or test aimed at improvement
  - Develop hypotheses or predictions
- Do
  - Carry out the change or test
  - If possible, plan small-scale tests or experiments
- Study
  - Assess results
  - Examine what you learned
  - Determine what went wrong
- Act
  - Adopt the change or abandon the plan
  - Initiate the cycle again

Use of the PDSA process is advantageous for the following reasons.

- It is widely used and accepted in healthcare.
- It is intuitive.
- It can be implemented rapidly across the organization.
- It is compatible with and supports the use of rapid cycle testing (RCT) (Langley et al. 1996).
- It promotes "process thinking" among staff.

Use of the PDSA process is disadvantageous for the following reasons.

- It relies heavily on intuition and tribal knowledge.
- It typically focuses on small projects and thus achieves minimal results.
- It rapidly hits a level of diminishing returns. Many healthcare organizations already have exhausted gains from PDSA.
- It does not employ a robust set of statistical tools.
- It lacks a strong accountability system that ensures implementation.

Lean Methodology and the Toyota Production System

Many attribute the origins of today's Lean concepts to two sources. The first is Toyota, which began a quest to improve the efficiency of its manufacturing plant after World War II. The second is a physicist named Eli Goldratt, whose work provided a rich conceptual framework for understanding bottlenecks and constraints limiting productivity. Lean methodology includes a variety of tools that help eliminate unnecessary steps and waste in processes, including categories of waste, value stream mapping, push-pull systems, and concepts of mistake proofing (Zidel 2006). Lean methodology:

- is intuitive;
- can be implemented rapidly with moderate training;
- does not rely on extensive data analysis;
- promotes process thinking among staff; and
- provides a rich theoretical context for examining patient flow.

Like PDSA, Lean methodology relies heavily on tribal knowledge and lacks statistical and analytical tools that assess variation.

Six Sigma Methodology

The goal of Six Sigma is to satisfy customer expectations. At the heart of Six Sigma is the recognition that every work process has variation that can cause a defect or service failure. *Six Sigma* is a statistical term used to measure the degree of variation or deviation from the average. The science of Six Sigma can be traced back to Motorola, where an engineer named Bill Smith adopted the name Six Sigma to characterize a set of tools for reducing harmful variation in work processes. By the mid-1990s, a host of large organizations, such as General Electric, Sun Microsystems, and other *Fortune* 500 companies, had integrated Six Sigma into their work (Caldwell, Brexler, and Gillem 2005).

Six Sigma has evolved into a rich amalgamation of proven quality tools and statistical science. It contains tools for organizing project improvement work, analyzing problems, generating ideas, testing solutions, and implementing controls to maintain gains.

The use of Six Sigma includes the following benefits.

- It provides a rich statistical tool set for understanding the harmful effects of variation.
- It provides a strong framework for building a business case for change and measuring return on investment.
- It includes robust tools to promote interdepartmental collaboration and improve departmental handoffs.
- Its techniques in regression analysis allow the identification of constraints and opportunities with statistical certainty.
- It provides excellent tools for hardwiring and retaining gains.

Some disadvantages to the use of Six Sigma follow.

- The process is prone to overanalysis or "analysis paralysis."
- The process is resource intensive.
- The process can slow speed to action and progress.
- The tool requires a Black Belt (a highly trained individual) to implement changes.

- Industrial jargon can be confusing and can discourage clinical staff.

Any discussion of Six Sigma involves the topic of DMAIC. DMAIC stands for Define, Measure, Analyze, Improve, and Control. It is the central platform for managing Six Sigma projects. The rigor of DMAIC attracts many to Six Sigma. Unfortunately, the speed of the industrial DMAIC model is also a source of its main weaknesses. Senior executives attest that the methodical DMAIC process can be slow to produce results.

The case of 3M, a company known for its innovation and prolific development of new products and markets, illustrates the risks of introducing industrial Six Sigma. In 2000, 3M recruited James McNerney from General Electric for chief executive officer. He announced that he would "change the DNA of the place" and introduced industrial Six Sigma. 3M realized some immediate gains in productivity and cost position, but other unintended changes smothered 3M's culture of innovation. Art Fry, the inventor of the Post-it note, blames 3M's recent lack of innovative sizzle on Six Sigma (Hindo 2007). The classic DMAIC process has paralyzed many healthcare organizations when form becomes more important than function and the value of analysis trumps speed and innovation.

A typical Six Sigma DMAIC project starts with a meeting to announce the chartering of a new project. Process owners and those involved in the project discuss data needs and the business case and rationale for the project. The meeting adjourns with the expectation that the designated quality professional (Black Belt) will conduct analysis and report findings to the group. Data are collected and analyzed over one to three months. During this time, the team waits for analysis and makes no implementations or changes. An appropriately scoped DMAIC project can take between four and six months, which means the team spends up to 50 percent of the time preparing to take action.

When the Black Belt presents the analysis, there likely will be additional questions and requests for more analysis, which may delay implementation further. The team remains entrenched in the Analyze phase and risks advancement to the Improve and Control phases.

Classic industrial DMAIC stems from the assumption that no action should be taken until the critical aspects of the problem are identified and fully analyzed because department managers are unable to identify bottlenecks through inherent knowledge and experience alone. However, groups of clinical managers and departments are rarely without ideas. Most teams are quick to identify issues and even offer possible solutions. Some teams already have numerous theories about what will improve the hospital's performance. There is a reasonable probability that if the team selects three or four projects on the basis of tribal knowledge alone, they will select at least one critical variable that will improve the process. As senior leaders, we must ask what value there is in delaying implementation when a team has ample opportunities to improve performance.

One alternative that can achieve speed to action without compromising the value of identifying the drivers of quality is to combine the effective components of Lean methodology and Six Sigma. Using Lean methodology, teams can start improving processes through RCT. At the same time, they can start analysis using the full depth and scope of Six Sigma to prepare for when they will search and be ready for new insights. The power of adopting this modified DMAIC approach to drive the speed of results is illustrated in Figures 6.1 and 6.2.

Figure 6.1 Traditional DMAIC Framework

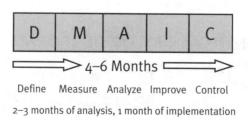

Define   Measure   Analyze   Improve   Control

2–3 months of analysis, 1 month of implementation

Figure 6.2 Accelerated DMAI²C Framework

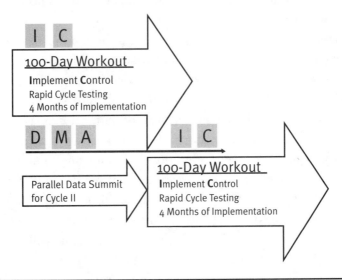

Use of this approach includes the following benefits.

- It removes the possibility that raising more questions about the data can delay implementation further.
- It provides three to four months of dedicated implementation time while data are being analyzed.
- It creates the expectation that implementation will commence regardless of the data process.
- It allows teams to exhaust their current ideas through RCT, which improves their receptivity to the Six Sigma analysis when it becomes available.

MAINTAINING A SET OF PERFORMANCE IMPROVEMENT TOOLS

When considering the best method for your organization, the optimal approach is to think of performance improvement as an evo-

What Top-Performing Healthcare Organizations Know

lutionary process in which all the tools are helpful at some point in the journey. Organizations naturally progress from using PDSA to using Lean methodology because PDSA is an excellent foundation for the acceleration tools of Lean methodology. Hospitals using Lean methodology quickly exhaust tribal knowledge and naturally introduce Six Sigma's rich statistical tool set to maintain momentum. As previously mentioned, organizations should consider using Lean methodology and Six Sigma as an inseparable set of tools. Both are valuable and serve different purposes.

Discarding one quality improvement method in favor of another generally is counterproductive. It sends a confusing message to staff and diminishes future progress. Staff will view new tools as the "flavor of the month" rather than a natural progression in the hospital's skill set. The best strategy is to maintain a robust set of tools and use the best method for each project. The best method will achieve the desired results with the least amount of effort in the shortest amount of time.

RESPONDING TO THE CHARACTERISTICS OF THE TEAM

Every team chartered for performance improvement starts from a different point, which alters the advanced quality methods likely to yield the most gains in the allotted time. Some teams are ready to initiate improvements, whereas others are approaching burnout. Senior executives can use the following framework to identify the qualities of a particular performance improvement team and determine which methods will work best.

- *Eager beavers.* This group is enthusiastic, biased toward action, and ready to change its work processes. The team is rich with testable ideas and strategies and has gathered the relevant inputs for change. To delay action when dealing with eager beavers would be a waste of time and would hamper progress. This group is willing to implement its ideas. Eager beavers should be moved into RCT as soon as possible. This group also may find PDSA helpful. Imposing the rigors of the classic DMAIC process on such a team may damper enthusiasm and delay results.

- *War horses.* This group is ready and willing to change but is searching for fresh insights. It has exhausted all known opportunities. Its current efforts are producing minimal performance gains, and there is a risk that further efforts will lead to frustration and diminishing returns. This group may benefit from a thorough analysis before initiating action. Six Sigma may be appropriate for this group.
- *Ostriches.* This team resists change and protects the status quo. A group may resist change because it has not experienced success with previous changes or is unconvinced of the need to change. More insight is needed to determine the appropriate quality method for this group. Leaders must determine the primary cause of its outlook. If the team is unconvinced of the need for change, an in-depth analysis and benchmarking may be required to support the opportunity for gain. If fear of failure or change is the barrier, moving directly into RCT may be the most appropriate course of action.

STRATEGIES FOR ACQUIRING EXPERTISE AND TOOLS

Many senior executives struggle with the best strategies for acquiring the skilled people necessary to implement quality improvement tools. Hospitals have three main strategies for developing the internal expertise required to support such methods:

- Hire a person from the manufacturing industry
- Hire a professional currently working in healthcare
- Develop talent internally

Each of these approaches has its own set of strengths and weaknesses.

Strategy 1: Hire an Expert from Manufacturing

Early adopters of advanced quality methods had few alternatives other than to hire candidates from the manufacturing industry. These experts were grounded in the application of industrial concepts as they apply to cost recovery and brought a fresh perspective to healthcare processes.

This strategy was not without challenges. These manufacturing experts faced learning thousands of acronyms and healthcare terms. Astute new employees needed months or years before they could communicate credibly with the medical staff. Sometimes physicians' multiple roles as customer, stakeholder, and process owner confused those unfamiliar with healthcare. For example, understanding the relationship between physician and hospital executive can be difficult for those uninitiated in healthcare.

In addition, healthcare's improvement opportunities reside in places different from those found in manufacturing and other industries. An expert from manufacturing may be highly experienced in reducing inventory, work in progress, and waste materials, whereas the healthcare industry's largest opportunities are in improving information and patient flow.

Today there are more industrial candidates with five or more years of healthcare experience. These candidates have spent the time necessary to clear the learning curve, learn the language of healthcare, and gain knowledge about the typical workflows of hospital departments. Senior leaders must remember that industrial thinking dominates these candidates' training in advanced quality methods. The traditional Lean-Six Sigma training does not include RCT, accountability structures, knowledge of healthcare information systems, or a strategic framework for achieving Big Q results. Despite these candidates' technical experience, senior leaders can expect to spend time coaching and creating a bias toward action and innovation.

Strategy 2: Hire an Expert from Healthcare

Today there are many candidates with training and experience in applying advanced quality methods, such as Lean-Six Sigma principles, to healthcare. A candidate with previous healthcare experience likely understands healthcare's unique language, culture, and major care processes. This experience even may accelerate the process of introducing new concepts to the organization.

However, external candidates will face the challenges of any other new employee. They will have to learn how to navigate the hospital's culture and build trust and credibility. Their job responsibilities will put them in the difficult role of meddler in the departmental operations of their peers.

When selecting an expert from within the healthcare field, senior leaders must identify candidates who have a demonstrated history of tangible results and who use tools that fit the circumstances rather than approach projects with a "one size fits all" strategy. External hires should not assume that solutions they implemented at other organizations will transfer to a new facility.

Strategy 3: Promote and Certify Current Employees

Experience has shown that developing internal talent through apprenticeship is the best approach for incorporating acceleration tools into an organization. These candidates already know the organization and its work processes. They understand its culture and have credibility with their peers. These factors are critical because technical skills are secondary to the candidate's ability to lead change and get things done.

Training internal candidates allows senior executives to shape their quality system from the beginning and avoid pitfalls and mistakes that commonly occur with an outside candidate. For example, senior executives can establish from the beginning the preferred methods of maintaining speed to action and avoiding excessive data analysis. They can establish their own agenda of introducing the organization to new methods and tools. Training of internal candidates can be paced to match organizational needs.

Internal candidates will need apprenticing and support to be successful in their new roles. When selecting internal candidates for advanced training, search for employees who have a bias toward action and know how to get things done. When facing a choice between a candidate who is highly analytical and a candidate who can organize teams and lead them to action, err on the side of the person who is action oriented. Remember that initiatives seldom fail during the analysis stage. Failure generally occurs at the start of implementation.

Apprenticeship Versus Training

Apprenticeship is the superior approach to developing internal candidates. Apprentices can directly observe the quality improvement tools being applied in their organization. Direct observation creates a rich learning environment that classroom training cannot replicate. The mentor or coach—such as a Master Black Belt in Six Sigma—can coach the candidate through inevitable barriers.

Senior leaders should encourage spaced repetition training and education that allows candidates the time to absorb and develop competencies with the methods. The traditional approach to training requires candidates to absorb a tremendous amount of technical information in a short amount of time. Spaced intervals of training allow candidates to develop competencies with each tool before moving on to the next.

Organizations should use public training courses as a last resort. Many public courses are industrially oriented or too generic to be applied to healthcare. They also do not provide candidates with the support necessary to develop in-depth knowledge of how to apply the tools in their specific organizations. Candidates are left on their own to translate these methods into approaches that work in healthcare.

"JUST IN TIME" TRAINING FOR MANAGERS

The successful introduction of any quality acceleration method requires a cultural shift in the way the organization views its work. Do not expect a team of two or three quality method experts, such as Six Sigma Black Belts, to evangelize the entire organization. A quality professional is seldom in a position to make department managers act. The quality professional only can support the identification of opportunities for improvement and make progress visible to executive leaders.

For these reasons, plan for the introduction of new quality methods to managers who must implement change. Individuals need not be trained to a uniform level of expertise, but everyone responsible for managing departments or developing staffing plans should be familiar with Lean concepts and categories of quality waste, and appreciate the role variation plays in quality.

When introducing new tools to managers, incorporate a practicum. A practicum ensures that participants develop a working knowledge of how to use the new methods to solve real problems, and it establishes an expectation that participants use the methods to achieve a tangible result. The practicum could take place during the 100-Day Quality Workout kickoff. During this time, quality professionals should present only the information and tools the managers will require to complete the next project. Quality professionals should avoid the temptation to overload managers with knowledge they will not apply immediately.

When training managers on advanced quality methods, quality professionals should create simplified templates and use healthcare terms and examples instead of method jargon.

CONCLUSION

Advanced quality methods can help organizations increase the speed and magnitude of their results when applied in the proper context.

Such tools are the third part of an organization's balanced approach to performance improvement, which includes an accountability system and an environment conducive to change. Senior leaders must ensure these methods are applied in a manner that promotes a bias toward action and innovation if rapid gains are to be maintained.

REFERENCES

Bradbury, I. 2008. "The Evolution of Deming's PDSA Cycle." [Online information; retrieved 3/4/08.] http://deming.ces.clemson.edu/pub/den/deming_pdsa.htm.

Caldwell, C., J. Brexler, and T. Gillem. 2005. *Lean-Six Sigma for Healthcare: A Senior Leader's Guide to Improving Cost and Throughput.* Milwaukee, WI: Quality Press.

Hindo, B. 2007. "3M's Innovation Crisis: How Six Sigma Almost Smothered Its Idea Culture." *Business Week* (June 11).

Langley, G. J., K. M. Nolan, I. W. Nolan, C. L. Norman, and L. P. Provost. 1996. *The Improvement Guide.* San Francisco: Jossey-Bass.

Zidel, T. 2006. *A Lean Guide to Transforming Healthcare: How to Implement Lean Principles in Hospitals, Medical Offices, Clinics and Other Healthcare Organizations.* Milwaukee, WI: Quality Press.

Seven Steps from Theory to Results

Your success in life isn't based on your ability to simply change. It is based on your ability to change faster than your competition.
—Mark Sanborn

THE AMERICAN COLLEGE OF HEALTHCARE EXECUTIVES developed this chapter as part of a course called "Aggressively Improve Costs and Throughput Using Lean Six Sigma" (Caldwell 2008). It is a guide to implementing the methods discussed in the previous chapters. It is organized as a seven-step approach to managing change initiatives in healthcare organizations and incorporates the research, concepts, and recommendations we have proposed for creating a unified system. Contained within each section are helpful questions designed to prompt strategy discussions among senior leaders and guide you through the process. By following the seven-step model, you can fully integrate your operational and quality/performance improvement strategies into a multiyear plan and move the organization swiftly into action.

1. Select a Big Q core process and metric that have the most impact on strategic and operational plans.
2. Assign accountability to the executive champion and key resources.

3. Prioritize sub-processes that drive Big Q goals.
4. Charter 100-Day Quality Workout projects based on identified sub-processes.
5. Track project milestones within the 100-Day Quality Workout structure.
6. Hardwire gains and charter the next 100-Day Quality Workout cycle project aimed at Big Q sub-processes and metrics.
7. Repeat these steps for the next Big Q core process.

STEP ONE: SELECT A BIG Q CORE PROCESS

The goal of step one is to achieve clarity of focus by having senior leadership establish the organization's Big Q core processes vital to success and determine the sequence in which Big Q Core processes will be addressed. By selecting one of these Big Q core processes as the focus of a performance improvement project, you are linking strategy to quality effectively.

To start this process, we suggest that senior teams achieve consensus and formally identify their Big Q core processes. This task will take some discussion, but the team must develop a unified sense of the core processes vital to the organization's performance. This step is key to achieving the focus required to implement meaningful change. When determining the Big Q core processes, keep the following points in mind.

- Identify your Big Q core processes and consolidate where possible. Refer to the definitions and questions in Chapter 4 as a litmus test of the strategic importance of the process.
- Use the suggested Big Q core process list found in Chapter 4 as a starting point for discussion. Modify as necessary. Limit the list of Big Q Core processes to no more than seven. Remember that focus is a vital element of success. Resist the temptation to dilute your list.

- Continue to test the suggested processes against the definition of a Big Q core process from Chapter 4. Are they strategic enough to warrant senior leaders' continuous attention? Are they large and important enough that we should be working on them continuously to make improvements?
- Establish effective process metrics. Avoid using averages. Instead, focus on establishing metrics that define quality and identify points at which patients/customers are repelled. For example, a goal can be stated as, "No patient entering the emergency department will wait more than 30 minutes to see a physician."

After achieving consensus on your Big Q Core processes, determine which one to focus on first. What is the most important improvement you can make in the next 100 days? The following questions can be useful as discussion guides when prioritizing your effort.

- Which Big Q core process provides the best opportunity to make strategic performance improvements in the next 100 days?
- Which process is within the organization's ability to execute and will bring about the most significant change?
- Which process will have the most impact on your strategic and operational goals?
- Where will gains in waste elimination and patient capacity produce tangible revenue?
- Where will gains in satisfaction improve patient market share, reduce recruiting costs, or produce other benefits?

STEP TWO: ASSIGN EXECUTIVE CHAMPION AND KEY RESOURCES

Step two addresses ownership of the key roles in managing a 100-Day Quality Workout (each of these roles is outlined in detail in Chapter 3). First, someone on the senior leadership team must fulfill the role of executive champion. If ownership at the senior leader level is not important to you, you have not selected a core process that is large or strategic enough. If you encounter resistance to senior leader ownership, consider going back and reviewing step one. You also should assign the other key roles to all performance improvement projects: workout coordinator, finance liaison, and communications coordinator. Depending on the scope and sophistication of the selected focus, you also may need to enlist a technical expert, such as a Six Sigma Black Belt or Lean professional. Use the following questions to guide your selections.

- Executive champion
  - Who will speak for the senior team?
  - Which senior leader would be the best owner of this core process and the results of the improvement effort?
  - Who has the positional authority and clout to remove obstacles to change and align incentives for interdepartmental collaboration?
  - Who can devote 8 to 12 hours per month to leading this 100-Day Quality Workout?
- Workout coordinators
  - Which staff members have strong organizational skills and reputations for getting things done?
  - Who have a passion for improving the organization's work and are not full-time managers?
  - On whom can the executive champion rely to be observant during the process?
  - Which individuals have the flexibility to commit 2 days per month to the 100-Day Quality Workout?
- Finance liaison
  - Which individual in the finance department is approachable and can build a working relationship with departmental managers?
  - Does this person have access to the hospital's financial and accounting information and expertise in cost accounting?
  - Who is best suited to assist managers in estimating the

tangible value of implemented or proposed changes to work processes?

- Does the candidate have enough experience to understand the concepts of the Big Q processes and the impact they will have on the hospital's performance?
- Can the candidate devote 1 to 2 days per month in support of the 100-Day Workout?
- Communication coordinator
  - Which candidate understands the message senior leaders want to deliver to the staff?
  - Who can develop an integrated communication plan for the hospital's quality system?
  - Who can translate the information obtained during manager meetings into effective communication pieces?
  - Who has the creative talent to help the executive champion plan and execute the celebration that occurs during the summation?
  - Can the candidate dedicate 1 to 2 days per month to the 100-Day Quality Workout?
- Technical quality/performance improvement expert
  - Will the hospital require extensive Lean or Six Sigma tools to complete the focus of the 100-Day Quality Workout?
  - Will managers and team leaders require technical support to drive change successfully?
  - Who will be responsible for providing the tools and training required to achieve the hospital's goal?

STEP THREE: PRIORITIZE SUB-PROCESSES THAT DRIVE BIG Q GOALS

Further refine your performance improvement focus by drilling down to specific sub-processes. For example, emergency department (ED) length of stay and 2 p.m. discharge are too large and complex to solve in 100 days. You may need to complete several successive

100-Day Quality Workouts to optimize these core processes. Select a maximum of three or four key sub-process drivers. For example, assume your team has selected the Big Q core process of patient flow through the ED. Even though you have determined that a reduced length of stay would demonstrate improvement in patient flow, do not assume that you can improve every aspect of the ED that affects length of stay in the next 100 days. Determine the sub-process drivers that have the greatest impact on ED length of stay.

At this juncture, senior leaders face a critical decision. They must determine whether extensive analysis using Six Sigma methodology will be required to identify these critical drivers or whether tribal knowledge will suffice to move ahead. Remember that we are inclined to collect more data and perform additional analyses. Most teams, however, can initially make progress through use of tribal knowledge and Lean tools. As a starting point for discussion, refer to the list of sub-processes you developed in Chapter 4. These sub-processes usually make the list and are a great place to start in the absence of a complete regression analysis of your facility. To retain your speed to action and eliminate needless delays in implementation, refer to the section on accelerated DMAI^{2}C and the differences in work teams outlined in Chapter 6.

Consider the following points when selecting sub-processes.

- Review the sub-process metrics in Chapter 4.
- Which sub-processes are likely to play a role in your facility?
- Which sub-process offers the highest probability of producing significant gains in the next 100 days?
- Do you have a strong understanding of your workflow process, and have you created a workflow map?
- Do the staff members involved in the work process understand the larger goal and their roles in the workflow process you have selected? Review Chapter 6.
- Does the team have sufficient tribal knowledge to take action and make progress? Are the managers replete with ideas and

strategies, or have they exhausted their current efforts? What is the starting point for the managers involved in making the proposed changes? Will additional data spur the team to action or cause further delays?

- If you achieve the desired improvement in quality and performance, what tangible gains and return on investment can you expect? Where will there be cost recovery?
- What resources and time commitment will be required to make the desired changes? Who (e.g., managers, process owners) will be involved in the changes? Do these individuals have the time to commit to the project? If not, how can capacity for change be created through reprioritization or a list of projects that are no longer useful?
- What is your capacity for change, and how many initiatives can the organization support at once? How much overlap is there among performance improvement initiatives?
- Are there activities or initiatives you should put on your list of unproductive projects or that you should suspend during the next 100 days to free up your capacity for change? Which nonstrategic projects can you eliminate?

You may think you need to analyze more data before you can determine the appropriate sub-processes on which to focus. However, you should resist the temptation to gravitate toward this assumption. If you have actionable information and insights, there is little value in delaying action. When you have exhausted actionable information, Lean-Six Sigma can be valuable. Regression analysis will assist you in identifying your critical focus areas.

Remember that some ambiguity and uncertainty always will be present. Keep team members focused on what they do know and what they can do. You can start today while you charter additional data analysis in preparation for the next cycle of improvement.

Consider the following questions when deciding whether to take action or engage in further data analysis.

- Does the team already have consulting reports, best practice recommendations, or internally generated strategies on which they can act?
- Has the team exhausted its ideas, and is further action unlikely to produce significant gains?
- Will additional analysis move the team to action or present only additional information to consider?
- Are there items the team can begin implementing while additional data are collected and analyzed?

If you require additional statistical analysis, your performance improvement experts should conduct a rapid assessment of the sources of necessary data and expected outcomes of the data analysis process. Formal training in quality improvement tools such as Lean-Six Sigma is valuable in such an assessment.

Generally, you should use Lean-Six Sigma's statistical methods to ascertain where to focus the improvement effort after you have addressed all actionable information. Lean tools provide a rapid start but will soon exhaust tribal knowledge. Before you run out of ideas, we recommend having a Lean-Six Sigma Black Belt download data from legacy information technology systems or initiate manual data sampling to run process capability and regression analysis to identify your critical focus areas. Review this information with the executive champion and key process owners (department managers). From this set of key drivers, you can determine areas of focus for the 100-Day Quality Workout, establish goals, and identify process owners who will drive the changes. Having selected critical sub-work processes, you can easily determine which managers will participate. This procedure is referred to as the *data summit process*. Consider the following questions when engaging in this activity.

- What data will be required? Can the desired data be pulled from the existing legacy IT systems to track a patient through the system?

- What resources, barriers, and priorities will you need to alter to make this analysis available?
- Who will be responsible for ensuring completion of these key tasks by the desired dates?

Once you have selected a sub-process on which to focus, determine the reaction you anticipate from staff. The question is not *whether* hospital employees will raise concerns, but rather *when* they will raise them and *what types* of concerns they will raise. One way to anticipate these reactions and develop a coordinated response is to determine main communication points for the project. Keep the following points in mind during this process.

- What is the appropriate response to questions from the senior leadership team?
- Is your message and response based on a quality message, or does it place cost and financial considerations first? Remember that staff will be less resistant to a quality-based message.
- What metrics do you hope to improve, and how much improvement do you expect? Have you articulated how you will measure the performance success of your work processes?
- What are your strategies, methods, and tools for communicating the appropriate message?
- What are the key communication points of your message for each stakeholder group?
- How will you know that the message points are effective and well received?

STEP FOUR: CHARTER A 100-DAY QUALITY WORKOUT

You have reached the point of moving the team into action. The 100-Day Quality Workout is our recommended structure for an accountability system. It has proven itself a reliable method for leading change and improving accountability across an organization. Think of the 100-Day Quality Workout not just as a project, but rather a cyclical quality system. When the current 100-Day Quality Workout ends, the next 100-Day Quality Workout is launched. Remember that whether you will be working on improving your processes is not in question. The only question is on what process you will focus. Creating these multiyear sequences increases your probability of achieving significant improvements in your Big Q goals.

After completing steps one through three, you have all the information you need to schedule dates for the kickoff of the next 100-Day Quality Workout. When setting up the workout, consider the following questions.

- Are you likely to complete this work in one 100-Day Quality Workout, or will you require a series of 100-Day Quality Workouts to complete your goal?
- What additional knowledge and skills will participants need to implement changes during this 100-Day Quality Workout? What apprenticing and training will be required during the two-hour education session and practicum? Who will be responsible for developing the content of the session and providing the technical support? What approach will you deploy to ensure that managers apply the tools in everyday work?
- Which managers and personnel will participate in the 100-Day Quality Workout?
- Which of your existing meetings, work teams, initiatives, or projects could you incorporate into the 100-Day Quality Workout structure?

Establish key dates. Instead of scheduling meetings around the calendars of individual participants, let the process drive the calendar to prevent slippage. Select dates for the following events:

- Kickoff (one day)
- 30-, 60-, and 90-day check-ins (two hours each)
- Summation (includes the kickoff of the next 100-Day Quality Workout) (one day)

People respond best when the desired result has been stated explicitly. Results seem to correlate with expectations set by the senior executive. For this reason, senior leaders should consider developing a vision statement for the workout. It can take the form of an inspirational challenge that sets expectations for all participants. This statement should be brief and concise, and clearly indicate leadership's expectations. Keep the following points in mind as you develop this statement.

- What challenge will senior leadership issue to the staff? Remember that research indicates quantum improvers emphasize activity goals rather than financial goals.
- What is the best way to state the challenge (e.g., number of successful changes accomplished, financial gains, achievement of full-time equivalent [FTE] targets, increases in patient flow or capacity)?

STEP FIVE: TRACK PROJECT MILESTONES WITHIN THE 100-DAY QUALITY WORKOUT STRUCTURE

The senior leadership team must achieve consensus on how it will track the sum of its performance improvement initiatives. We recommend having a central platform for entering projects and updating results. Without a centralized inventory, assessing progress will be difficult. The senior team should consider the following questions when creating this inventory.

- By what tool or method will we make progress visible?
- Is our tool simple enough for every manager to use with minimal training or instruction?
- What is the basic set of information we require managers to enter?
- At what point of detail will the tracking become onerous and complicated and produce diminishing returns?
- On what physical platform will the tracking system reside (e.g., Word documents, Excel spreadsheets, project management software, legacy systems, Internet- or intranet-based applications)?

STEP SIX: HARDWIRE THE GAINS AND CHARTER THE NEXT 100-DAY QUALITY WORKOUT

By the time you reach step six, the staff has completed changes in work processes and produced tangible gains. Senior leaders must recognize that vigilance is not a quality system and is doomed to failure. You cannot rely on human attention to hold gains indefinitely. Gains rapidly dissipate unless senior leadership makes a deliberate effort to build belief in the change and hardwire the gains into the culture and work processes. Momentum also must be maintained once progress has been achieved.

Industrial engineers and Lean experts use engineering concepts to design an error-free process. Likewise, we have identified 84 change concepts that include design principles such as visual cues, forcing functions, and standardization. These 84 concepts are a composite list of process engineering strategies for hardwiring change. Seventy-five of the change concepts come from page 295 of *The Improvement Guide* (Langley et al. 1996), and we added eight as a result of our work in the field. (A copy of the list of 84 change concepts can be downloaded at www.chipcaldwellassoc.com.) By verifying that solid design principles have been applied, senior leaders can avoid Kotter's (1995) error 7, declaring victory too soon, and error 8, not anchoring changes in the corporation's culture.

To hardwire gains and continue momentum, senior leaders should ask the following questions at the 30-, 60-, and 90-day check-ins.

- What methods will we use to build belief in the changes and to prevent returning to old patterns?
  - Are we using rapid cycle testing (RCT) to build belief in changes?
  - Do the implemented solutions appear to hospital staff as "home grown" or foreign solutions imposed by an external source?
- To retain the current gains, are teams using proven engineering concepts to prevent slippage?
  - Are teams and managers relying on vigilance or the design of work processes?
  - Have we developed detection and control plans and implemented them to trigger remedial action if there is slippage?
- What is the appropriate focus of the next 100-Day Quality Workout?
  - What steps are required to introduce the next focus?
  - What actions do we need to initiate today to be prepared to kick off the next 100-Day Quality Workout?
  - What data and analysis will we require?
  - What training and new methods will we require for managers to be successful?

STEP SEVEN: REPEAT THE PROCESS

Step seven is about maintaining momentum and continuity. We recommend that the executive champion maintain a plan that specifies the order and focus of the 100-Day Quality Workouts, and review and prioritize it on a regular basis with the senior team.

FROM UNDERSTANDING THE STEPS TO REAL-WORLD APPLICATION

To help you visualize the application of the seven-step process, the following case studies illustrate its application in three organizations, focusing on different aspects of their operations.

Case Study One: 400-Bed Facility Facing Increasing Competition

Situation
A 400-bed community hospital located in the Southwest was enjoying a strong, growing market and healthy operating margins. The CEO was concerned that the hospital staff had become complacent after 30 years of prosperity. He knew the hospital needed to prepare for increasing competition and market pressures that would force the organization to be more efficient. However, he was concerned that staff would perceive initiatives to improve performance as cost cutting and not support them, given the hospital's strong financial condition.

Solution

Step 1: Select a Big Q Core Process
To preserve operating margin, the senior team decided to declare war on all forms of quality waste. It announced that this decision was part of a broader initiative to improve the organization's ability to serve the community by using its resources wisely. The net benefit would be increased patient flow, reductions in wait times, and the ability to deliver more care to the community. It also announced that it expected patient and physician satisfaction to improve as a result of these efforts.

Step 2: Assign Accountability to Executive Champion and Key Resources
The CEO appointed the chief operating officer (COO) as executive champion and appointed others to fill the key roles of finance

liaison, workout coordinator, and communication coordinator. The COO began working with his team on a communication strategy to impart a quality message assuring all stakeholders that they were launching this initiative out of a genuine desire to improve quality and performance and not as a veiled cost-cutting effort. They named the program "Journey to Excellence."

Step 3: Prioritize Sub-Processes That Drive Big Q Goals

Senior leaders announced that the hospital's initial focus would be the elimination of the seven categories of waste from all departmental processes. Senior leaders were concerned that establishing financial benchmarks would corrupt the spirit of the initiative. Instead, they chose to establish metrics based on the number of changes each manager was required to make. In this case, each manager was required make a minimum of two changes per month, or eight changes in the next 100 days.

Step 4: Charter 100-Day Quality Workout Projects Based on Identified Sub-Processes

In previous years, the hospital had suffered from starting and stopping programs. The senior team was concerned that staff would perceive a new initiative as another "flavor of the month." There also had been a movement to bring collaboration and forms of shared governance into the hospital. The team thought that the 100-Day Quality Workout structure would serve as a clearinghouse for the exchange of ideas and a way to track the progress of each workgroup. The senior team communicated the following points to the organization.

- The hospital always will be engaged in performance improvement.
- Three cycles of improvement will be conducted per year, focused on strategies determined by the senior leadership team.
- Meetings will be set on a fixed day every month, and participation will be mandatory.

- Many existing teams will be folded into this structure.
- This initiative will be part of a longer journey toward embracing Lean-Six Sigma. New tools will be introduced during each cycle.

Step 5: Track Project Milestones Within the 100-Day Quality Workout Structure

Senior leadership anticipated that managers would claim they were too busy with existing initiatives to participate. The senior leadership team proactively responded by requiring the use of an Internet-based tracking tool for all performance improvement efforts. Their goal was to take an inventory of all the hospital's initiatives and develop with the managers a list of projects that are no longer useful. This action allowed them to free up resources and send a clear message that they were serious about measuring progress.

Step 6: Hardwire Gains and Charter the Next 100-Day Quality Workout Cycle

The managers identified $7.5 million in potential gains and realized approximately $6.1 million during the first 100 days of the program. The finance liaison reviewed each idea to validate that the savings from the change were real and to determine whether the gain would be recurring. An industrial engineer monitored the managers' work to see that they had taken appropriate steps to hardwire the changes in the work process.

Step 7: Repeat Steps for the Next Big Q Core Process Until a Steady State Is Achieved

This hospital is in its seventh 100-Day Quality Workout cycle, focusing on core processes such as in-quality staffing, ED length of stay, 2 p.m. discharge/60 minutes to next patient, and surgery cut-to-close. During each of these 100-Day Quality Workouts, selected staff members were certified in Lean-Six Sigma to sustain the organization's efforts and achieve self-sufficiency. During the first year, the hospital recovered $11.5 million in annualized gains.

Case Study Two: 300-Bed Hospital Facing Staffing Challenges

Situation

A 300-bed community hospital located in the Southeast was facing increasing budget pressures. State Medicaid cuts and changes in payer mix threatened to consume the hospital's margins. As a result, senior leadership had no choice but to initiate layoffs, hiring and salary freezes, and across-the-board budget cuts. These changes restored the hospital to profitability and allowed it to regain a solid financial footing. However, the hospital is located in a very close community, and there were the predictable side effects of layoff, including reduced trust of staff and backlash from the community and physicians.

Following the layoffs, the team initiated a program called OPI (operational performance improvement). In its first year, the program was successful and generated just under $5 million in additional cost recovery. In the subsequent year, the OPI program saw diminishing returns and generated less than $1 million in gains despite considerable efforts. Managers were convinced that no more gains could be realized, and the program stagnated.

They knew they needed to find a way to reinvigorate their efforts and help their staff find new methods of improving performance. As a result, they chartered an initiative focused on the elimination of quality waste in the organization. The senior team introduced managers to Lean methodology's seven categories of waste and discussed the 84 change concepts with them to ensure that they had incorporated engineering principles into their work process designs. During the first 100-Day Quality Workout, the organization successfully recovered $5.8 million in tangible cost, as reviewed by the finance liaison.

Senior leaders also knew they still had opportunity to improve their staffing patterns. They thought about using a standard benchmarking approach to staffing but were fearful of manager backlash to the external productivity targets. They also wanted to avoid intimation of a slash-and-burn approach to FTEs.

Solution

Step 1: Select a Big Q Core Process

The senior team wanted to use a quality-based approach to the staffing issue and selected the in-quality staffing approach as its next focus. When staff members raised concerns that another round of layoffs might be imminent, the senior team was able to point to the steps of this approach and assure them that quality was at the root of the initiatives. First, the senior team communicated that managers would set the definition of quality. Second, decisions would be made on the basis of their data. Third, managers would develop an ideal staffing plan. Fourth, managers, with their vice presidents, would establish the implementation plan and timetable for changes. The team also reminded managers that the process would identify understaffing just as well as it would identify overstaffing.

Step 2: Assign Accountability to Executive Champion and Key Resources

The CEO appointed the COO as the executive champion and appointed others to fill the key roles of finance liaison, workout coordinator, and communication coordinator.

Step 3: Prioritize Sub-Processes That Drive Big Q Goals

The senior team started the revitalization process by challenging department managers with aggressive benchmarks that demonstrated the hospital had approximately $12 million in opportunity. The $12 million figure resulted from moving the hospital's performance from the 50th percentile to the 75th percentile. The CEO made a preemptory strike on staff concerns by stating that the hospital was still doing well and the "best time to change is before we have to." The CEO asked the staff to close half the performance gap during the next 120 days. He clearly communicated that this directive was not about working harder but working smarter and changing work processes. To accomplish this goal, each manager was provided an overview of the in-quality staffing process and trained in a process that included five steps:

- Establishing each manager's definition of in-quality staffing
- Collecting hourly data on staffing levels and demand
- Developing the ideal staffing plan
- Developing a plan for transforming the current plan into the ideal staffing plan
- Implementing changes and RCT

Step 4: Charter 100-Day Quality Workout Project Based on Identified Sub-Processes

The team used the 100-Day Quality Workout to drive accountability and created the following timeline.

- Kickoff—Managers complete training on in-quality staffing process and tools.
- 30-day check-in—Managers present data and analysis outlining how current staffing matches their definition of quality.
- 60-day check-in—Managers have developed their ideal staffing plan and identified potential solutions to improve staffing. Implementation of RCT is initiated.
- 90-day check-in—Managers continue making changes and improving the percentage of time they meet their definition of quality staffing.
- Summation—Managers confirm plans for hardwiring the changes and protecting the gains.

Step 5: Track Project Milestones Within the 100-Day Quality Workout Structure

Senior leadership had all participants track their progress using an Internet-based tool that made results visible to the entire organization. In addition to monitoring progress, leadership used this tracking tool in other notable ways:

- To inspire competition for ideas and results among similar nursing units and ancillary departments

- To challenge managers who already had met their goal to explore other change categories and strategies (e.g., if a manager had achieved results using three of the eight change concepts, the challenge was to implement additional changes incorporating at least two more change concepts)

Step 6: Hardwire Gains and Charter the Next 100-Day Quality Workout Cycle

The managers identified $3.5 million in potential gains and realized approximately $2.1 million during the first 100 days of the program. They accomplished these gains through a variety of means. Several units created formal attrition plans. Other units eliminated the burden of minimum staffing and variation in patient census by establishing "sister units," which resulted in a new wave of cross-training and job sharing that increased flexibility in responding to variations in demand. This process produced additional gains by reducing the use of agency nursing. By examining their patient demand on an hour-by-hour basis, units were able to identify predictable patterns and adjust their staffing plans accordingly. These units were able to implement irregular shifts and stagger 12-hour shifts to match staffing with demand.

Step 7: Repeat Steps for the Next Big Q Core Process Until a Steady State Is Achieved

This hospital went on to charter a 100-Day Quality Workout Cycle focused on ED length of stay and patients left without treatment. The CEO decided that each senior leader would own at least one Big Q core process. He determined that the senior staff member in the role of executive champion would change according to the focus of the 100-Day Quality Workout. His decision communicated that everyone on the senior team owned part of the quality system and would be involved in improving performance.

Case Study Three: 450-Bed Metropolitan Hospital Facing Long ED Length of Stay

Situation

A large medical center in Florida was under increasing pressure to reduce wait times in its ED. Senior leaders recognized that conventional "silo" approaches to quality improvement would exhaust the organization. Attempts to form multidisciplinary taskforces and committees had failed to produce results. Prior initiatives were continuously derailed by the next daily crisis. Furthermore, the team was involved in a perpetual debate about which solutions would be best for the ED. A new idea and solution were always right around the corner. Senior leaders knew the only way to achieve progress was to create a structured approach toward testing changes and direct all their energy toward implementation.

Solution

Step 1: Select a Big Q Core Process

The senior team chose ED length of stay and reduction of patients left without treatment as the strategic focus for the next 100 days. The ED's goal was to admit patients in less than four hours or discharge them in less than three hours. Currently, the hospital was measuring only the average ED wait times, which indicated that it was approximately three hours. Staff believed that this three-hour standard was acceptable on the basis of the community's expectation. However, after looking at the variation in ED length of stay, the process capability analysis indicated that the ED was achieving its definition of quality less than 60 percent of the time. Therefore, 40 percent of ED visits resulted in lengths of stay that exceeded the three-hour average.

Step 2: Assign Accountability to Executive Champion and Key Resources

The COO appointed the chief of nursing as executive champion and appointed others to fill the roles of finance liaison, workout coordinator, and communication coordinator. Senior leadership expressed that physicians should be informed and involved in the initiative where appropriate. Meetings were scheduled to communicate the intent of the ED initiative to key individuals. During these meetings, an overview of the initiative's processes and safeguards was provided to demonstrate that changes would be tested and not decrease the quality of care or service levels.

Step 3: Prioritize Sub-Processes That Drive Big Q Goals

Before starting the initiative, a data summit and an analysis of the ED's data were conducted to identify the ED's capacity constraints. The data summit connected all the hospital's legacy systems and departmental data into a comprehensive data set. From this data, a regression analysis was completed that pinpointed the ED's top constraints as:

- last lab to ED discharge;
- last radiology to ED discharge;
- triage to ED bed;
- first radiology order to last verified; and
- ED bed to physician assessment.

On the basis of this analysis, five multidisciplinary teams were assembled to tackle these areas. Each team had to make at least two successful changes in work processes within the next 100 days. The goal was to find solutions to eliminate the harmful variation in work processes that blocks patient flow. Each team worked on a specific aspect of ED flow and shared results with the other teams to produce harmonious solutions.

Step 4: Charter 100-Day Quality Workout Project According to Identified Sub-Processes

The senior team elected to use the 100-Day Quality Workout structure and thought that monthly reporting of results and progress by all teams would harness positive peer pressure and generate momentum. By the 60-day check-in, all the teams had produced demonstrable results and implemented at least one successful change. For example, employees realized that although bed request processing took two hours, they could initiate the process sooner. Data indicated that within five minutes of seeing a patient, physicians knew with 90 percent accuracy whether the patient would be admitted and what type of bed he or she would require. This change in thinking allowed the staff to move from a linear process to a parallel process that greatly reduced delays in transferring patients out of the ED. Initially, the team believed that success depended on quicker turnaround of lab test results. Data indicated that waiting for physicians to respond to the patient's last lab test produced the delays. As a result, design changes were made to the information system and presentation of information to physicians that allowed them to respond to results faster. The key to progress was having the team test its ideas. Apprenticing in Lean-Six Sigma, RCT, and the 100-Day Quality Workout gave the team the knowledge it needed to perform these tests.

Step 5: Track Project Milestones Within the 100-Day Quality Workout Structure

Senior leadership communicated that milestones would be tracked and published for the organization. At each check-in, the communications coordinator captured notes from the reports and formatted the information for various stakeholders. At the completion of the 100-Day Quality Workout, the organization published a newsletter describing the results of each change and rapid cycle test. By publishing this newsletter, senior leaders reemphasized their intent to make progress visible.

Step 6: Hardwire Gains and Charter the Next 100-Day Quality Workout Cycle

The teams tested and implemented changes that reduced the average length of stay by 2.5 hours. These changes resulted in an estimated $4.2 million in additional revenue and gains in productivity. The Master Black Belt and Black Belt candidates designed control steps modeled on Lean-Six Sigma methods and the 84 change concepts to hardwire the changes into the ED workflow.

Step 7: Repeat Steps for the Next Big Q Core Process Until a Steady State Is Achieved

This hospital developed a robust quality system as staff members evolved into Master Black Belts in Lean-Six Sigma. Senior leaders used their experience in the ED to charter two additional 100-Day Quality Workouts to improve the 2 p.m. discharge metric and increase quality waste recovery. The 100-Day Quality Workouts provided staff the opportunity to apply quality acceleration methods like Lean-Six Sigma and, more important, changed the culture to foster inter-departmental collaboration rather than department-specific activity. The process enhanced relationships among ED staff; ED physicians; hospitalists; and bed management, discharge planning, transport, housekeeping, lab, imaging, and inpatient unit personnel. As a result of these efforts, the hospital increased its bottom line by more than $7 million in the first two 100-Day Quality Workouts and improved customer mandates for more efficient, speedier patient flow through the organization. Application of Lean to quality waste recovery in the third 100-Day Quality Workout recovered an additional $3.1 million.

REFERENCES

Caldwell, C. 2008. "Aggressively Improve Costs and Throughput Using Lean Six Sigma." Seminar presented by American College of Healthcare Executives, Keystone, CO, January 30–31.

Kotter, J. 1995. "Leading Change: Why Transformational Efforts Fail." *Harvard Business Review* 73 (2): 59–67.

Langley, G. J., K. M. Nolan, I. W. Nolan, C. L. Nolan, and L. P. Provost. 1996. *The Improvement Guide*. San Francisco: Jossey-Bass.

Afterword

THERE IS A SAYING that a smart man learns from his mistakes, but a wise man learns from the mistakes of others. We sincerely hope that you profit from the lessons that formed the basis of this book. Driving meaningful change in healthcare is a complicated business, but the pathways to success tend to take a simple form. We witnessed this book's techniques save hundreds of millions of dollars in healthcare costs when senior leaders implemented these solutions as a comprehensive quality system instead of focusing on training alone. We saw self-acknowledged nonstarter hospitals transform themselves into quantum improvers in less than 100 days by simply backing their efforts with the proper structure for transforming their care processes. Our experience continues to demonstrate that the structure of transformational initiatives is the most critical variable in achieving meaningful progress and predicting success.

These findings place senior leaders in control of their destiny. Taking steps to design a structure of accountability, create an environment of change, and develop a strategic framework that focuses the organization on the right issues will help you break the status quo and gain momentum. Once these elements are in place, tools such as Lean-Six Sigma will accelerate the pace of change if appropriately adapted to the healthcare environment.

Today is the time for you to design your quality system. We encourage you to embrace the methods presented in this book and adopt them as your own. Using the guiding principles we outlined, you can modify your program over time to fit the culture of your organization. To aid you in this process, we summarized points worth remembering.

POINTS WORTH REMEMBERING

1. Senior leaders must take ownership of their quality system and keep it at a strategic level.
2. Senior leaders must be comfortable coaching the larger aspects of quality.
3. The organization must establish a strong accountability system and environment of change. Be mindful that all advanced quality methods such as Lean and Six Sigma have proven minimally effective unless deployed in the right structure.
4. Design an environment of change that celebrates calculated risk taking, innovation, and failure that leads to progress. Conversely, the environment should make managers who protect the status quo uncomfortable. Focus on positive peer pressure and minimize negative peer pressure in your design.
5. Create organization-wide focus by developing your own list of Big Q Core processes, and maintain strategic focus by linking all performance improvement activities to these processes. Avoid delegating projects and resources down to the department level, where you lose the ability to drive significant improvements. Remember that you will realize your most significant gains when you focus your efforts on the handoffs between departments.
6. Organizations that focus their efforts on improving one or two large core processes at a time for brief periods tend to produce better results than organizations that dissipate

their efforts across a large number of projects spread across the entire hospital. Think strategic focus versus a bucket of projects.

7. Senior leaders must end the arguments over which advanced quality tool is best. You eventually will need Lean-Six Sigma and other advanced quality methods. Each contains tools for specific jobs, just as a hammer, screwdriver, and saw are used for specific jobs.

8. Advanced quality tools such as Lean-Six Sigma will accelerate your results when coupled with a strong accountability system and environment for change.

9. Introducing Lean or Six Sigma as an exercise in training alone will set you up for failure and result in minimal performance gains. Training and certification are only the start. Quantum improvers approach the application of knowledge systematically.

10. Remember that quantum improvers focus on creating a bias toward action. Always design your quality system and tools accordingly. Avoid letting traditional benchmarking and classic Six Sigma approaches slow your organization's progress. Whenever possible, use acceleration methods and techniques such as the gap closure method of goal setting, rapid cycle testing, and accelerated DMAI^{2}C.

11. Insist that your performance improvement staff reduce or eliminate the unnecessary industrial jargon of Lean and Six Sigma. The direct application of manufacturing terms has proven to be less effective because it turns off healthcare professionals and hinders progress. For example, you do not need a lesson on Japanese to incorporate elements of Lean or the Toyota Production System, nor do you need to spend time educating staff on Six Sigma terms such as *defects per million opportunities*. Instead, make a conscious effort to translate the jargon into terms that fit your culture and embrace the language of healthcare.

12. Sustain your gains by designing a quality system that builds belief in change through repeated experience. Rapid cycle testing is an excellent tool for this purpose. In addition, take steps to ensure engineering design principles are incorporated into the changes to eliminate reliance on human vigilance.

13. Create a tracking system for all your performance improvement initiatives. It will help make progress visible across the organization. In addition, it will allow the senior team to better manage the organization's capacity for change and create a list of projects that are no longer useful.

14. If a performance improvement initiative is important enough to commit resources to, it is important enough to have a formal communication plan. A sustained communication effort should be in place before the launch of any major initiative.

15. Maintain the integrity of your quality system by incorporating mechanisms that track tangible financial gains. Whether the goal is improving patient satisfaction, clinical outcomes, or patient flow, always expect a return on investment. If you are eliminating waste, errors, delays, and other impediments to quality, there should be tangible cost recovery. Insist that every quality professional in the organization be assigned an annual return on investment to be validated by your finance department. Expect a 5:1 return as a general guideline. Demand it, measure it, and track it relentlessly. If the quality professionals are not producing this level of return, consider them overhead.

Anyone who tells you that leading transformational efforts in healthcare is easy is surely inexperienced or misguided. Breaking down the status quo is not a business for the weak. If success were all just about the vision, personal charisma, or organizational culture, a leader's capacity to influence the outcome would be limited to his or her ability. Instead, we should be inspired by findings that indicate success is influenced more by variables we can directly manage and influence. The tangible way in which transformation efforts are organized plays the greatest role in predicting the success of any project. There are steps you can take as a senior leader to increase your probability of success and improve the sustainability of your gains. Creating a structure that imbeds these principles appears to trump the intangible side of culture.

As healthcare professionals, researchers, and authors, we remain dedicated to assisting the healthcare industry in its application of advanced quality methods. If you would like to review additional case studies or download copies of the tools presented in this book, visit the website listed below.

If you are interested in having your organization participate in good-to-best research or want to learn more about ongoing research on attributes of quantum improvers, access the website listed below and click on "Quantum Improver Assessment 360 Survey." As a participant, you will receive valuable insight on how you can optimize your organization's quality system. For more information on this project, contact us at:

Chip Caldwell & Associates
P.O. Box 3273
St. Augustine, Florida 32085-3273
www.chipcaldwellassoc.com
(832) 372-2465

As authors, we welcome your feedback and suggestions. We also appreciate opportunities to learn from your experiences as you implement the concepts presented in this book. We wish you the best of luck in your journey.

About the Authors

Greg Butler is executive vice president of Chip Caldwell & Associates and brings more than 25 years of experience to leading change and innovation in the healthcare industry. During his career, Greg has held leadership positions with some of the country's leading healthcare manufacturers, consulting firms, and healthcare service providers. Greg served as senior vice president for Cardinal Health Clinical Consulting & Services, vice president of marketing and business development for Owen Healthcare, and senior director for VHA/Novation.

For the past 15 years, Greg has assisted hospitals in improving productivity, patient flow, and pharmacy operations and lowering operating costs. This work includes developing strategies for applying advanced quality methods to common needs such as reducing emergency room overcrowding, expanding operating room capacity, minimizing length of stay, and improving patient satisfaction and clinical utilization. Greg is a certified Green Belt in Lean-Six Sigma. He holds an MBA from the University of Texas at Dallas and a BBA from Texas Tech University.

Chip Caldwell, FACHE, is president of Chip Caldwell & Associates and considered a thought leader in healthcare quality and performance improvement methodology. For the past decade, he has been a leader in the quality community, serving as a member of the Baldrige Foundation Board Support Team and a healthcare representative on the U.S. Quality Council, as well as with numerous organizations, including Premier Performance Services, Juran Institute, Atlanta Health System, and HCA West Paces Medical Center in Atlanta. His books are widely read by hospital board members, senior leaders, middle managers, and health administration students. Chip has extensive practical knowledge of hospital operations and is the leading executive faculty on the effective use of Lean-Six Sigma in healthcare for the American College of Healthcare Executives and the American Society for Quality (ASQ). Chip has trained over 10,000 executives in such prestigious organizations as IBM, Veterans Administration, PruCare, Kaiser, U.S. Navy, Premier, VHA, and ASQ.